# Emeril L
# Power Air Fryer 360 Cookbook 2022



*By David Martin*



**Warning-Disclaimer:**

The purpose of this book is to educate and entertain. The author or publisher does not guarantee that anyone following the techniques, suggestions, tips, ideas, or strategies will become successful. The author and publisher shall have neither liability or responsibility to anyone with respect to any loss or damage caused, or alleged to be caused, directly or indirectly by the information contained in this book.

# CONTENTS

# INTRODUCTION

## AIR FRYING BASICS

In the simplest of terms, an air-fryer is a compact cylindrical countertop convection oven. It's a kitchen appliance that uses superheated air to cook foods, giving results very similar to deep-frying or high-temperature roasting. Many of us have convection ovens in our kitchens. In a standard oven, air is heated and the hot air cooks the food. In a convection oven, air is heated and then blown around by a fan. This creates more energy and consequently cooks foods faster and more evenly.

Air fryers use the same technology as convection ovens, but instead of blowing the air around a large rectangular box, it is blown around in a compact cylinder and the food sits in a perforated basket. This is much more efficient and creates an intense environment of heat from which the food cannot escape. The result is food with a crispy brown exterior and moist tender interior – results similar to deep-frying, but without all the oil and fat needed to deep-fry. In fact, when you are air-frying, you usually use no more than one tablespoon of oil!

Better still, an air fryer doesn't just cook foods that you would usually deep-fry. It can cook any foods that you would normally cook in your oven or microwave as well. It is a great tool for re-heating foods without making them rubbery, and is a perfect and quick way to prepare ingredients as well as make meals. To me, it is the best new kitchen appliance that has been introduced in recent years.

## HEALTH BENEFITS

Obviously, because it can produce results similar to deep-frying using a tiny fraction of the oil needed to deep-fry, the health benefits are apparent. When deep-frying, you submerge the food in oil and oil is inevitably absorbed by the food. In an air fryer, you still use oil because oil is what helps crisp and brown many foods, but you really don't need more than one tablespoon at a time. Instead of putting the tablespoon of oil in the air fryer, you simply toss foods with oil and then place them in the air fryer basket. In fact, spraying the foods lightly with oil is an even easier way to get foods evenly coated with the least amount of oil. Investing in a kitchen spray bottle is a great idea if you have an air fryer.

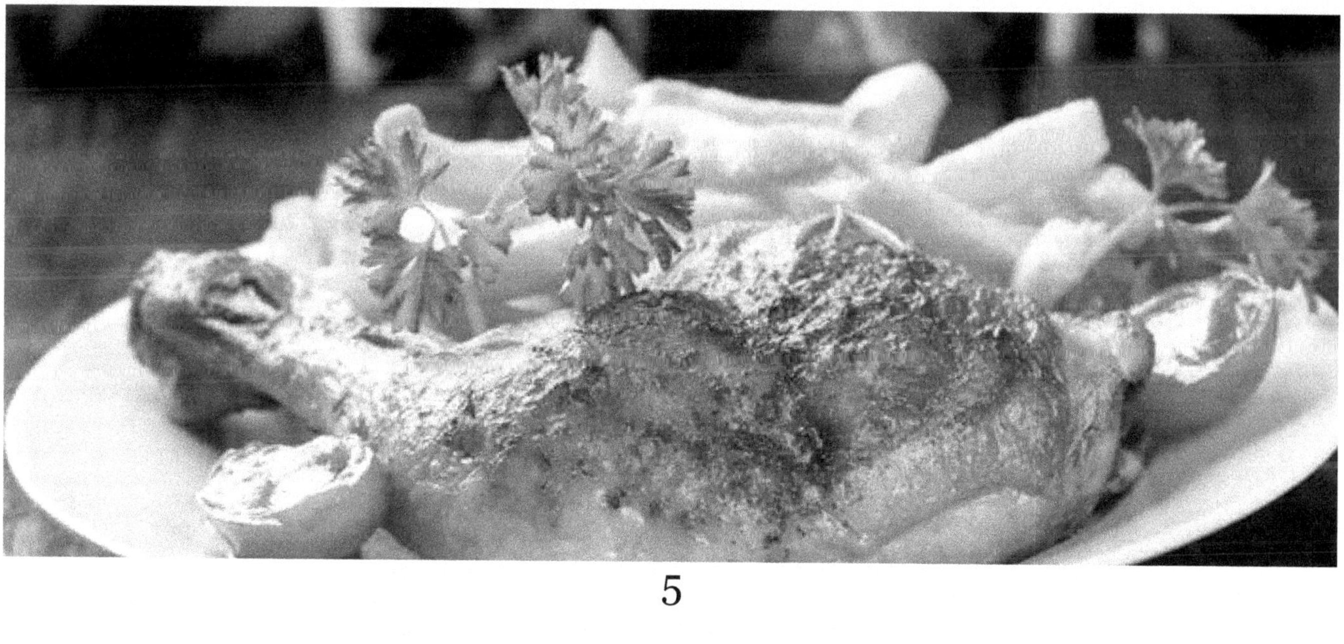

## QUICK AND ENERGY EFFICIENT

We all know that sometimes it can take fifteen to twenty minutes to pre-heat our standard ovens. Because the air fryer is so compact, that pre-heat time is cut down to two or three minutes! That's a huge savings in time as well as energy. In the summer, you can pre-heat your air fryer and not heat up the whole kitchen. In addition, the intense heat created in the air fryer cooks foods quickly, about 20% faster than in an oven, so you're saving time and energy there as well. No one these days seems to have time to spare, so this should please everyone!

## SAFE AND EASY TO USE

Air-frying is safer and easier than deep-frying. Most air fryers have settings for time and temperature. You simply enter both and press start. It doesn't get much easier than that! When deep-frying, you have to heat a large pot of oil on the stovetop, use a deep-frying thermometer to register the temperature and then monitor the heat below the pot to maintain that temperature. On top of it all, you are dealing with a lot of oil, which can be heavy to move, dangerous if it gets too hot, and is cumbersome and annoying to drain and dispose of. Why bother if you can get the same results so much more easily with an air fryer?

## CLEAN AND TIDY

I didn't earn the "Miss Tidy Bed" badge in brownies for no reason! I love keeping the kitchen clean and tidy when I'm cooking and after I've been cooking. The air fryer fits into my world perfectly. It cooks foods in a contained space and that keeps the food from splattering anywhere. Period. You can even cook bacon in the air fryer without making a mess (do remember the tip to put a little water in the drawer below to prevent the bacon grease from smoking). It is simple and straightforward to clean and keep clean, and you know what they say about cleanliness...

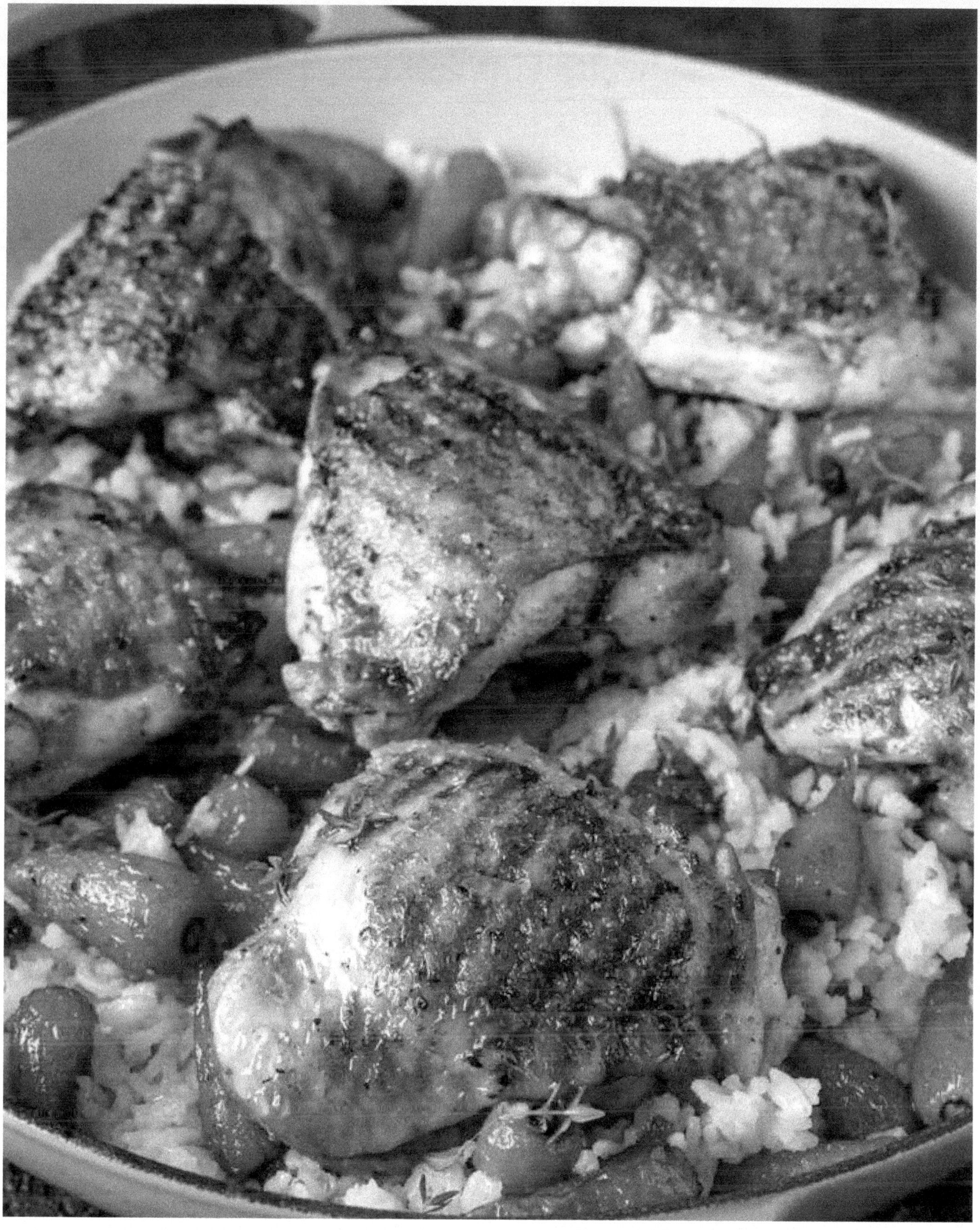

# OF OUR ABSOLUTE FAVORITE AIR-FRYER RECIPES TO TRY AT HOME

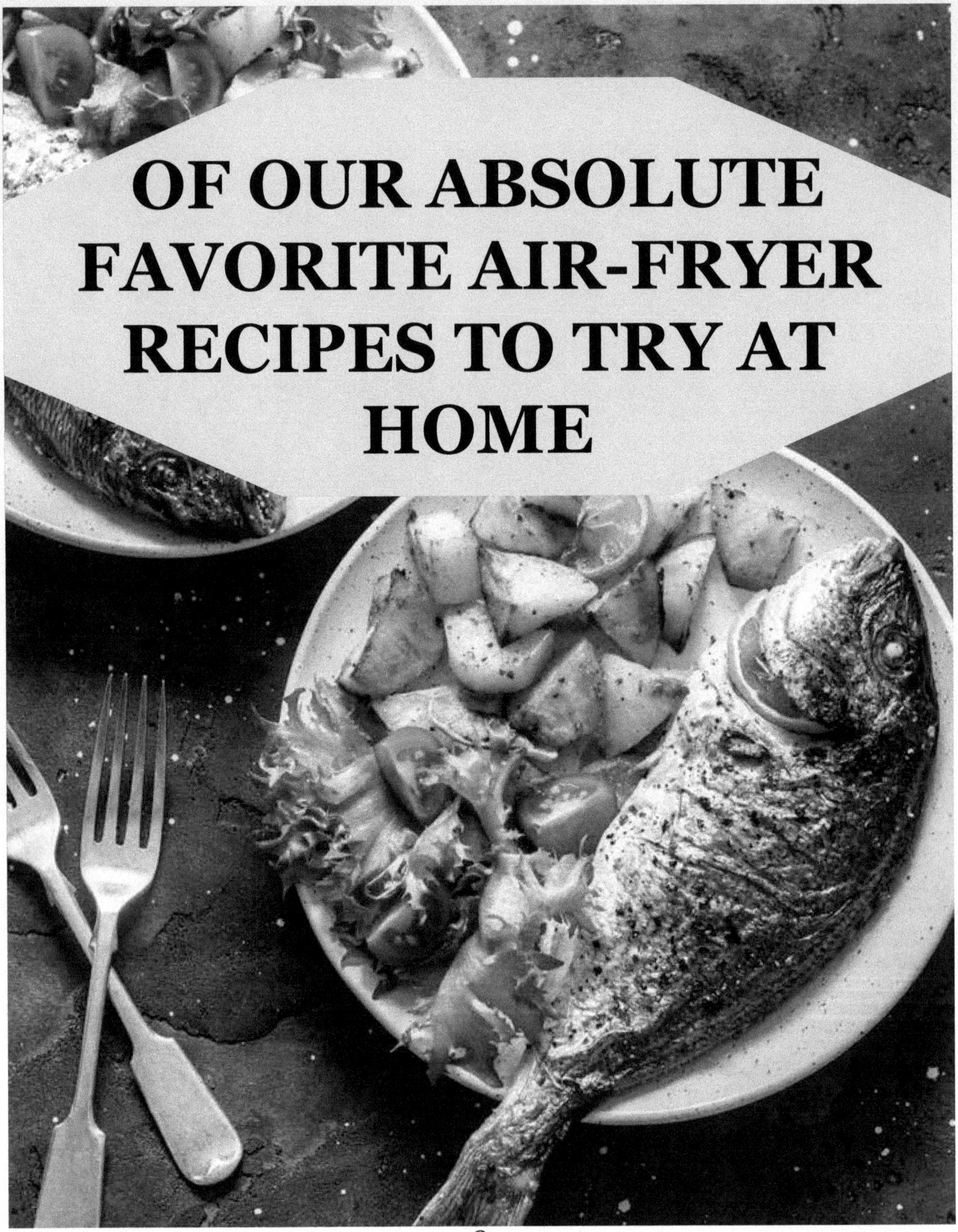

## Air Fryer Shrimp Fajitas

**Prep Time: 10 minutes** **Cook Time: 22 minutes** **Servings: 12**

### INGREDIENTS

- 1 Red Bell Pepper Diced
- 1 Green Bell Pepper Diced
- 1/2 Cup Sweet Onion Diced
- 2 Tbsp of Gluten-Free Fajita or Taco Seasoning
- 1 Pound Medium Shrimp Tail-Off (Cooked, Frozen Shrimp)
- Olive Oil Spray
- White Corn Tortillas or Flour Tortillas

### DIRECTIONS

1. Spray the air fryer basket with olive oil spray or line with foil.
2. If the shrimp is frozen with ice on it, run cold water over it to get the ice off.
3. Add the peppers, onion, and seasoning to the basket.
4. Add a coat of olive oil spray.
5. Mix it all together.
6. Cook at 390 degrees for 12 minutes using the air fryer or air crisp function of the Ninja Foodi.
7. Open the lid, and add in the shrimp for the final 10 minutes, spray it again, and mix it together.
8. Cook an additional 10 minutes.
9. Serve on warm tortillas.
10. This recipe uses cooked, frozen shrimp, it can be made with uncooked shrimp too but may need a few additional minutes of cook time.

## Honey Glazed Air Fryer Salmon

**Prep Time: 2 minutes** **Cook Time: 8 minutes** **Servings: 4**

### INGREDIENTS

- 4 Salmon Fillets , skin on (see note 1)
- Salt (see note 2)
- Black Pepper (see note 3)
- 2 teaspoons Soy Sauce (see note 4)
- 1 tablespoon Honey
- 1 teaspoon Sesame Seeds

### DIRECTIONS

1. Preheat the air fryer (mine takes 2 minutes).
2. Meanwhile: Season each salmon fillet with salt and pepper. Brush the soy sauce into the fish.
3. Place the fillets into the air fryer basket (skin side down) and cook them at 375°F (190°C) for 8 minutes or until ready.
4. About a minute or two before the time is up, glaze each fillet with honey and sprinkle with sesame seeds. Put them back in and finish cooking.
5. Serve with a side of your choice.

# Air Fryer Crab Rangoon

**Prep Time: 45 minutes** **Cook Time: 10 minutes** **Servings: 15**

## INGREDIENTS

- 30 Wonton Wrappers
- 7.5 oz Jalapeño Cream Cheese
- 6 oz Imitation Crab Meat chopped
- 2 tsp Soy Sauce
- 2 tsp fresh lemon juice
- 2 tbsp vegetable oil
- Duck Sauce

## DIRECTIONS

1. Soften the cream cheese.
2. In a clean bowl, stir together the cream cheese, soy sauce and lemon juice.
3. Fold in the chopped crab until well blended.
4. Using the photos as a guide, fill the wontons with the filling and fold. This recipe makes about 30 Crab Rangoon.
5. Cook the Crab Rangoon in batches in the air fryer. My basket holds about 8 at a time. There's no need to flip the Crab Rangoon.
6. Place the Crab Rangoon in the air fryer basket in a single layer. Brush each lightly with vegetable oil. Cook at 375 degrees F for 7-8 minutes. Until the Crab Rangoon are puffed and lightly brown.
7. Serve with Duck Sauce for dipping.

# Air Fryer Roasted Balsamic Brussels Sprouts

**Prep Time: 10 minutes** **Cook Time: 15 minutes** **Servings: 4**

## INGREDIENTS

- 1 pound brussels sprouts , ends removed and cut into bite sized pieces
- 2 Tablespoons olive oil , or more if needed
- 1 Tablespoon balsamic vinegar
- kosher salt , to taste
- black pepper , to taste

## DIRECTIONS

1. Put cut brussels sprouts to bowl. Drizzle oil and balsamic vinegar evenly over the brussels sprouts. Don't dump the oil and vinegar in one spot or else it will just coat one brussels sprout. You want to make sure to coat all the brussels sprouts.
2. Sprinkle salt and pepper evenly over the brussels sprouts. Stir to combine everything and long enough so that all the brussels sprouts soaks up the marinade. There shouldn't be any marinade left in the bottom of the bowl.
3. Add brussels to the air fryer basket. Air fry at 360°F for about 15-20 minutes. Shake and gently stir half way through, about 8 minutes into cooking. Make sure you shake at the halfway mark! You don't wany to end up with uneven cooking. If needed, shake and toss a 3rd time to make sure it all cooks evenly.
4. Continue to air fry the brussels for the remainder of the time, or until the brussels are golden brown and cooked through. You can check earlier if needed to make sure nothing burns. Or you can add more time if needed to make sure it's cooked through.
5. Add additional salt and pepper if needed on the brussels sprouts and enjoy!

## Air Fryer Pizza Sliders

**Prep Time**: **10 minutes** **Cook Time**: **5 minutes** **Servings**: **12**

### INGREDIENTS

- 12 Slider rolls 4 English muffins can be substituted
- 1/2 cup pizza sauce
- 12 slices provolone cheese
- 1/2 cup mozzarella cheese
- 2 ounces pepperoni
- 1 teaspoon Italian seasoning

### DIRECTIONS

1. Cover solid tray from toaster oven tightly with foil. Split Hawaiians nearly in half to make an open faced sandwich.
2. Spread pizza sauce on rolls. Add a layer of sliced cheese and then cover with additional shredded cheese if desired
3. Arrange pepperoni and other toppings on pizza sliders.
4. Sprinkle Italian seasong on top and bake for about 5 minutes at 350°F on the convection bake setting in an air fryer/toaster oven. Mini pizzas are ready when cheese is melted.

## Air Fryer Mac 'n' Cheese Balls

**Prep Time**: **15 minutes** **Cook Time**: **12 minutes** **Servings**: **16**

### INGREDIENTS

- Fried Mac and Cheese Ball Ingredients
- 4 cups (600g) leftover mac and cheese
- 2 eggs beaten
- 2 cups (300g) seasoned bread crumbs

### DIRECTIONS

1. Air Fried Mac and Cheese Balls Directions
2. To make your mac and cheese balls, start by chilling the leftover mac and cheese in your fridge for 3 hours.
3. Next, scoop out about 1 1/2 tablespoon of mac and cheese, roll it and form it into a ball. This should make about 16 mac n cheese balls.
4. Taking one mac and cheese ball at a time, dip and roll each ball in the egg and dredge it through the bread crumbs. Make sure the entire ball gets coated in bread crumbs. Continue with each ball until all of the macaroni cheese balls are covered.
5. Freeze the balls for 30 minutes while you preheat your Air Fryer to 360 F / 182 C.
6. Carefully place the mac and cheese balls in the Air Fryer, making sure that they don't touch each other. Fry for 10-12 minutes until golden. You don't need to worry about turning them halfway through. Depending on the size of your Air Fryer, this will probably need to be done in multiple batches.

# Air Fryer Churros

**Prep Time: 10 minutes Cook Time: 10 minutes Servings: 8**

## INGREDIENTS

- 1 cup water
- 1/3 cup unsalted butter cut into cubes
- 2 Tbsp granulated sugar
- 1/4 tsp salt
- 1 cup all-purpose flour
- 2 large eggs
- 1 tsp vanilla extract
- oil spray
- Cinnamon-sugar coating:
- 1/2 cup granulated sugar
- 3/4 tsp ground cinnamon

## DIRECTIONS

1. Put a silicone baking mat on a baking sheet and spray with oil spray.
2. In a medium saucepan add water, butter, sugar, and salt. Bring to a boil over medium-high heat.
3. Reduce heat to medium-low and add flour to the saucepan. Stirring constantly with a rubber spatula cook until the dough comes together and is smooth.
4. Remove from heat and transfer the dough to a mixing bowl. Let cool for 4 minutes.
5. Add eggs and vanilla extract to the mixing bowl and mix using an electric hand mixer or stand mixer until dough comes together. The mixture will look like gluey mashed potatoes. Use your hands to press lumps together into a ball and transfer to a large piping bag fitted with a large star-shaped tip.
6. Pipe churros onto the greased baking mat, into 4-inch lengths and cut end with scissors.
7. Refrigerate piped churros on the baking sheet for 1 hour.
8. Carefully transfer churros with a cookie spatula to the Air Fryer basket, leaving about 1/2-inch space between churros. Spray churros with oil spray. Depending on the size of your Air Fryer you have to fry them in batches.
9. Air fry at 375 degrees F for 10-12 minutes until golden brown.
10. In a shallow bowl combine granulated sugar and cinnamon.
11. Immediately transfer baked churros to the bowl with the sugar mixture and toss to coat. Working in batches. Serve warm with Nutella or chocolate dipping sauce.

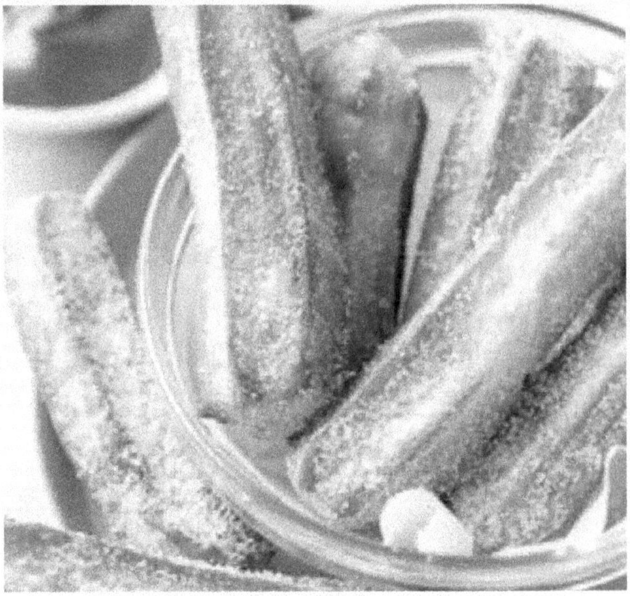

# Air Fryer Sesame Chicken

**Prep Time: 10 minutes  Cook Time: 25 minutes  Servings: 6**

## INGREDIENTS

### Chicken

- 6 Boneless Skinless Chicken Thighs
- 1/2 Cup Cornstarch
- Olive Oil Spray

### Sauce

- 1/4 Cup Soy Sauce or Gluten-Free Soy Sauce
- 2 Tbsp Brown Sugar
- 2 Tbsp Orange Juice
- 5 Tsp Hoisin Sauce or Gluten-Free Sauce
- 1/2 Tsp Ground Ginger
- 1 Garlic Clove Crushed
- 1 Tbsp Cold Water
- 1 Tbsp Cornstarch
- 2 Tsp Sesame Seeds
- Optional
- Green Onions
- Cooked Rice

## DIRECTIONS

1. Cut the chicken into cubed chunks, then toss in a bowl with Cornstarch or Potato Starch. Use enough to coat the chicken evenly.
2. Place in the Air Fryer and cook according to your Air Fryer Manual for chicken. (Note - I cooked ours on 390* for 24 Minutes, 12 minutes on each side.)When the chicken is in the air fryer, add a nice even coat of olive oil cooking spray, once it's in the air fryer, it works best to mix it up halfway through cook time and add an additional coat of spray.
3. While the chicken is cooking, in a small saucepan, begin to make the sauce.
4. Add the soy sauce, brown sugar, orange juice, hoisin sauce, ground ginger, and garlic to the saucepan on medium-high heat. Whisk this up until well combined.
5. Once the sugar has fully dissolved and a low boil is reached, whisk in the water and cornstarch.
6. Mix in the sesame seeds. (The sauce should only take about 5 minutes or less to make on the stove and then an additional 5 minutes to thicken up.)
7. Remove the sauce from the heat and set aside for 5 minutes to thicken.
8. Once the chicken is done, remove from the air fryer and place in a bowl, and then coat with the sauce.
9. Serve topped over rice and beans.

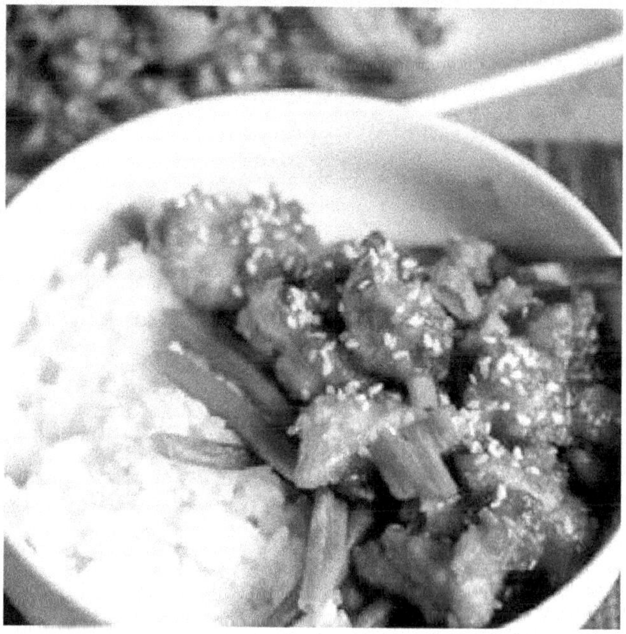

# Air Fryer Chilean Sea Bass

**Prep Time: 5 minutes   Cook Time: 20 minutes   Servings: 2**

## INGREDIENTS

- 2 6 ounce chilean sea bass fillets
- 1 tablespoon unsalted butter
- 1/4 cup white miso paste
- 1 tablespoon rice wine vinegar
- 4 tablespoons maple syrup, honey works too!
- 2 tablespoons mirin
- 1/2 teaspoon ginger paste
- olive oil for cooking
- fresh cracked pepper
- Optional toppings
- sesame seeds
- sliced green onions

## DIRECTIONS

1. Preheat air fryer to 375° F. Brush olive oil all over each fillet of fish and finish with fresh cracked pepper. Spritz the air fryer pan with olive oil and place the fish skin side down. Cook for 12-15 minutes, until the top begins to turn golden brown and the internal temperature has reached 135° F.
2. While the fish is cooking, melt the butter in a small saucepan over medium heat. When the butter has melted, add the miso paste, rice wine vinegar, maple syrup, maple syrup, mirin, and ginger paste. Stir until fully combined, bring to a light boil, and remove the pan from the heat immediately.
3. When the fish is finished, use a silicone pastry brush (or the back of a spoon) to brush the glaze over the top and sides of the fish. Place it back in the air fryer for 1-2 more minutes at 375° F, until the glaze caramelizes. Finish with sliced green onions and/or sesame seeds.
4. Oven Directions
5. Preheat the oven to 425° F and line a baking sheet with foil lightly sprayed with olive oil. Bake for 20-25 minutes, depending on the thickness of your fish. The internal temperature should be 135° F when the fish is cooked through.
6. Remove the fish from the oven and preheat the broiler to high. Brush the miso glaze over the fish (top and sides) and place it back in the oven on the top rack. *If your rack is too close to the broiler, move it down a bit, you don't want the fish to touch it!* Cook the fish for 1-2 minutes under the broiler, until it begins to caramelize. Keep a close eye on it because it happens quickly! Finish with sliced green onions and/or sesame seeds.

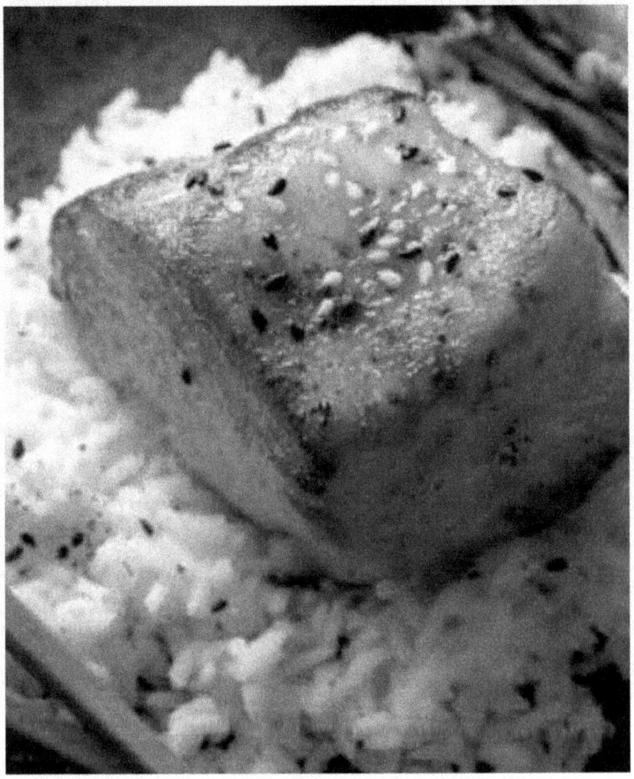

# Air Fryer Bang Bang Chicken

**Prep Time: 15 minutes** **Cook Time: 15 minutes** **Servings: 4**

## INGREDIENTS

**Bang Bang Chicken Sauce**

- 1/2 cup mayonnaise
- 2 tablespoons raw honey
- 1/2 tablespoon sriracha sauce or to taste
- Bang Bang Chicken Batter
- 1 cup buttermilk
- 2/3 cup all-purpose flour more if needed
- 1/2 cup cornstarch
- 1 egg
- 1 teaspoon sriracha sauce or to taste
- salt & pepper to taste
- 1 lb boneless & skinless chicken breast or chicken thighs - cut into bite size pieces
- 1 cup Panko bread crumbs more in needed
- oil of your choice for greasing air fryer

## DIRECTIONS

1. How to make Bang Bang Chicken Sauce
2. To make bang bang chicken sauce, combine all ingredients in a mixing bowl. Whisk until everything is combined. Set aside.
3. How to make Bang Bang Chicken in Air Fryer
4. To make bang bang chicken in air fryer, first make buttermilk batter by combining buttermilk, flour, corn starch, egg, sriracha sauce, salt and pepper. Then whisk until combined.
5. Grease Air Fryer with any oil of your choice before adding chicken. Next, working in batches, dip chicken pieces in buttermilk batter then breadcrumbs and add it into the Air Fryer. Air Fry at 375F for 8-10 minutes or until chicken is cooked thru. Flip the chicken pieces on the other side once. (Make sure not to crowd the chicken pices inside the air fryer.)
6. Drizzle the sauce over the chicken and serve with leafy greens or Fried Rice Recipe with Eggs and Green Onion. Enjoy!

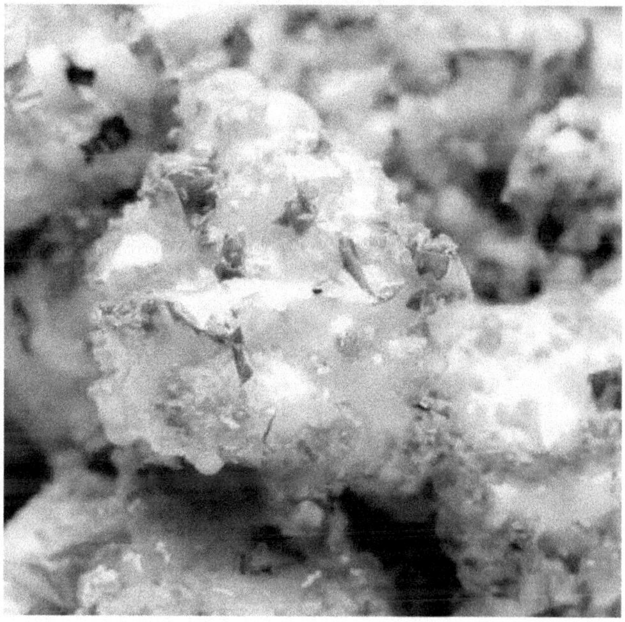

# Air Fryer Eggplant Parmesan

**Prep Time: 15 minutes Cook Time: 25 minutes Servings: 4**

**INGREDIENTS**

- 1 large eggplant mine was around 1.25 lb
- 1/2 cup whole wheat bread crumbs
- 3 tbsp finely grated parmesan cheese
- salt to taste
- 1 tsp Italian seasoning mix
- 3 tbsp whole wheat flour
- 1 egg + 1 tbsp water
- olive oil spray
- 1 cup marinara sauce
- 1/4 cup grated mozzarella cheese
- fresh parsley or basil to garnish

**DIRECTIONS**

1. Cut eggplant into roughly 1/2" slices. Rub some salt on both sides of the slices and leave it for at least 10-15 minutes.
2. Meanwhile in a small bowl mix egg with water and flour to prepare the batter.
3. In a medium shallow plate combine bread crumbs, parmesan cheese, Italian seasoning blend, and some salt. Mix thoroughly.
4. Now apply the batter to each eggplant slice evenly. Dip the battered slices in the breadcrumb mix to coat it evenly on all sides. See the helpful tips section above to do this task perfectly.
5. Place breaded eggplant slices on a clean and dry flat plate and spray oil on them. See notes section for details.
6. Preheat the Air Fryer to 360F. Then put the eggplant slices on the wire mesh and cook for about 8 min.
7. Top the air fried slices with about 1 tablespoon of marinara sauce and lightly spread fresh mozzarella cheese on it. Cook the eggplant for another 1-2 min or until the cheese melts.
8. Serve warm on the side of your favorite pasta.

◇◇◇◇◇◇◇◇◇◇◇◇◇◇◇◇◇◇◇◇◇◇◇◇◇◇◇◇◇◇◇◇◇◇◇◇◇◇◇◇

# Air Fryer Crispy Parmesan Cod

**Prep Time: 10 minutes Cook Time: 15 minutes Servings: 4**

**INGREDIENTS**

- 1 pound cod filets
- salt and pepper
- 1/2 cup flour
- 2 large eggs
- 1/2 teaspoon salt
- 1 cup Panko
- 1/2 cup grated parmesan
- 2 teaspoons old bay seasoning
- 1/2 teaspoon garlic powder
- olive oil spray if needed

**DIRECTIONS**

1. Salt and pepper the cod filets.
2. Create a breading station for the fish. In one bowl add the flour. In the second bowl whisk together the eggs and salt. In the last bowl add the Panko, parmesan cheese, old bay seasoning, and garlic powder.
3. First dip the cod in the flour.
4. Then in the egg mixture.
5. And lastly in the Panko.
6. Spray the bottom of your basket with olive oil. Place the fish in the basket of your air fryer. Cook at 400 degrees for 10 minutes. Carefully flip the fish. Continue to cook for 3-5 minutes or until the internal temperature reaches 145 degrees.

# Air Fryer Falafel

**Prep Time: 50 minutes Cook Time: 10 minutes Servings: 18**

## INGREDIENTS

**For the Falafel**

- 1 15 oz can chickpeas drained
- 1 cup chopped white onion
- 6 small cloves garlic
- 1 tablespoon lemon juice
- 1 cup lightly packed parsley leaves
- ½ cup lightly packed cilantro leaves
- ¼ cup lightly packed fresh dill leaves
- 1 teaspoon baking powder
- 2 teaspoons cuminutes
- 1 teaspoon salt
- ½ cup flour (either all-purpose flour or 1:1 gluten free flour)

**For the Vegan Yogurt Tahini Sauce**

- 1 cup vegan plain yogurt (not vanilla flavored)
- 1 tablespoons tahini (see notes)
- 2 tablespoons lemon juice

## DIRECTIONS

1. Add chickpeas, onion, garlic, lemon juice, parsley, cilantro, dill, flour, baking powder, cumin, and salt to a food processor. Pulse until a coarse crumb texture is formed. Stop to scrape down the sides of the bowl as needed.
2. Transfer the falafel mixture to a bowl, cover, and refrigerate for 1 hour (or up to 2 days before cooking).
3. While the falafel mixture sets, prepare the vegan tahini sauce. Whisk together the vegan yogurt, tahini, and lemon juice until combined. Add salt and pepper and stir to combine. Cover and refrigerate until time to serve.
4. Once the falafel mixture is chilled, use a spoon or cookie dough scooper to measure out 1 tablespoon of the dough. Form into balls. Place falafel balls on a plate. Repeat until all the batter has been used.
5. Spray the air fryer basket with vegetable cooking spray. Preheat air fryer to 375°F.
6. Use tongs to place raw falafel in the basket, arranging them on the bottom of the basket. Return basket to air fryer and cook for 15 minutes, removing the basket and using tongs to turn falafel once or twice during cooking time. Once done, remove falafel from the air fryer basket. Allow them to cool slightly.
7. To serve, place falafel on a plate and serve with tahini sauce for dipping. Or add 3–4 falafel inside a halved, pita along with hummus, chopped romaine lettuce, and chopped onions. Drizzle with the tahini sauce.

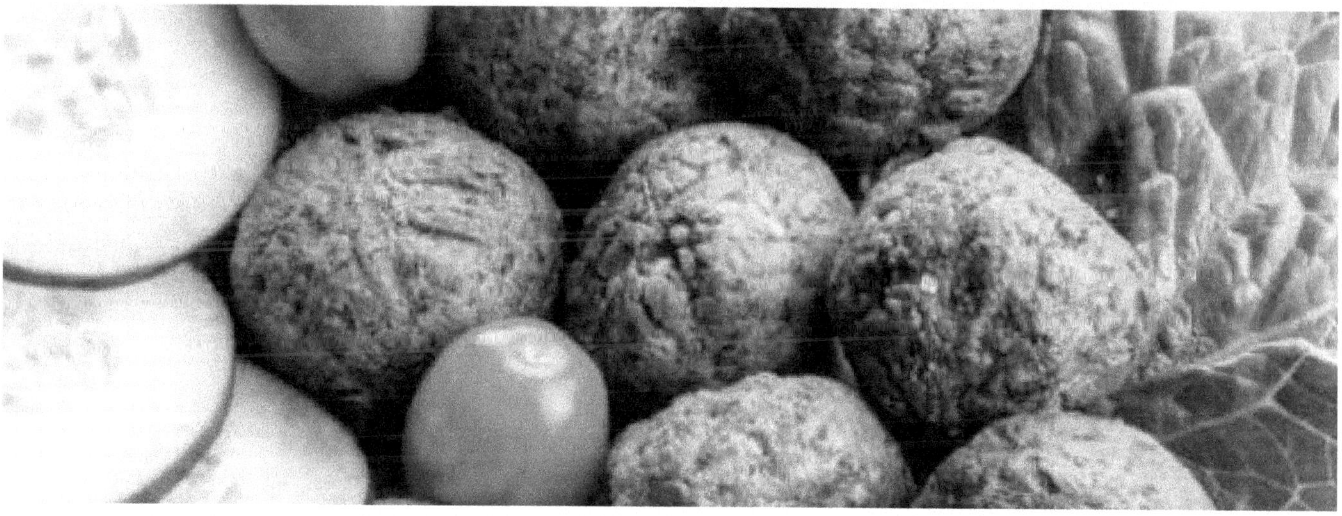

# Air Fryer Burgers

**Prep Time: 10 minutes    Cook Time: 12 minutes    Servings: 4**

### INGREDIENTS

- 1 lb ground hamburger recommend 85/15
- 1 tsp Worcestershire sauce
- 1 tsp seasoning salt
- 1 tsp garlic powder
- 1 tsp onion powder
- 4 slices cheese
- 4 buns
- *additional toppings like lettuce tomatoes, pickles, bacon ketchup, mustard. mayonnaise etc.

### DIRECTIONS

1. In a large mixing bowl combine hamburger, Worcestershire sauce, seasoning salt, garlic powder and onion powder and combine with hands. Do not overmix. Form into 4 patties.
2. Place the burgers in the air fryer, you may have to cook two at a time depending on the size of your air fryer.
3. Cook the burgers for 8 minutes at 360 degrees F. Flip the burgers over and cook for an additional 6-8 minutes or until the internal temperature of the burgers are 160 degrees F.
4. Top each burger with a slice of cheese and cook for an additional minute or until the cheese is melted.
5. Serve on buns with your favorite condiments.

◇◇◇◇◇◇◇◇◇◇◇◇◇◇◇◇◇◇◇◇◇◇◇◇◇◇◇◇◇◇◇◇◇◇◇◇◇◇◇

# Air Fryer Wonton Mozzarella Sticks

**Prep Time: 5 minutes    Cook Time: 6 minutes    Servings: 2**

### INGREDIENTS

- 6 mozzarella cheese sticks
- 6 egg roll wrappers
- olive oil spray
- kosher salt

### DIRECTIONS

1. 1. Place a piece of string cheese near the bottom corner of the egg roll wrapper. Roll up halfway and carefully fold the sides toward center over the cheese. Dip your finger in water and trace the edges of the wrapper. Roll the remaining wrapper around the mozzarella stick. Repeat with remaining wrappers and cheese.
2. 2. Place six of the mozzarella sticks in the air fryer and spray with olive oil spray. Sprinkle with kosher salt.
3. 2. Air fry at 350 degrees for 3 minutes, flip, spray the other side with olive oil spray and sprinkle with kosher salt, then continue cooking for another 3 minutes. Serve with marinara sauce for dipping, if desired.

# Crispy Air Fryer Corn Dogs

**Prep Time**: **10 minutes** **Cook Time**: **8 minutes** **Servings**: **8**

## INGREDIENTS

- 4 hot dogs (you can use beef hot dogs or turkey hot dogs)
- 3/4 cup yellow cornmeal
- 3/4 cup all-purpose flour (plus for more rolling)
- 1 ½ teaspoons baking powder
- 1/2 teaspoon baking soda
- 1 teaspoon sugar
- 1/2 teaspoon salt
- 3/4 cup buttermilk
- 2 eggs
- 1 ½ cups bread crumbs
- cooking spray

## DIRECTIONS

1. In a mixing bowl, whisk together cornmeal, flour, baking powder, baking soda, sugar, and salt.
2. In another bowl, whisk together buttermilk and eggs.
3. Add the buttermilk and egg mixture into the dry ingredients. Mix to combine. (Make sure there are no streaks of flour in the mixture.)
4. Transfer the batter to a tall glass. (Leave enough room to dip the hot dog without overflowing the glass.)
5. Pour the breadcrumbs in a bowl and set aside.
6. Cut the hot dogs (and the skewers) into halves, and skewer the mini hot dogs onto wooden sticks.
7. Roll the hot dogs in flour to coat, and shake off the excess.
8. Dip the floured hot dogs into the batter and then cover the battered hot dogs with breadcrumbs. Press the breadcrumbs onto the hot dogs gently using your hands.
9. Spray cooking spray on the hot dogs, and then place them in the basket in one layer. Make sure not to overcrowd your air fryer. Cook in batches if necessary.
10. Set the temperature to 375°F, and set the time to 8 minutes.
11. After 4 minutes, take out the basket and flip the corn dogs.
12. Return the basket to the air fryer. After 2 more minutes, check every 1 minute until heated through. Serve with ketchup and mustard if desired.

## Air Fryer Honey Sesame Salmon

**Prep Time: 5 minutes  Cook Time: 10 minutes  Servings: 4**

### INGREDIENTS

- 1 tablespoon sesame oil
- 1/4 cup honey
- 1 tablespoon sriracha
- 2 tablespoon soy sauce
- 3 cloves of garlic, minced
- Black pepper, freshly ground, to taste
- Salt, to taste
- 4 salmon fillets

### DIRECTIONS

1. In a small bowl, mix together ingredients 1-7 to make the marinade.
2. Put salmon fillets in a large bowl and pour half the marinade over them. Coat well.
3. Pre-heat air fryer to 375°F
4. Line air fryer basket with foil, and make some holes in the foil to match the air fryer basket holes (You could skip this step and just spray basket with cooking spray or use parchment paper liners with holes if you have them)
5. Transfer the salmon into the air fryer basket, making sure the fillets are not touching each other. Air fry for 8-10 minutes. Salmon is done when it flakes easily.
6. Meanwhile, pour the rest of the marinade into a small sauce pan and cook on stove over medium heat for a couple of minutes, until it thickens to form the glaze
7. When ready to serve, transfer salmon to plate and brush with glaze and sprinkle with chopped green onions and sesame seeds (optional).
8. Best served warm.

◇◇◇◇◇◇◇◇◇◇◇◇◇◇◇◇◇◇◇◇◇◇◇◇◇◇◇◇◇◇◇◇◇◇◇◇

## Air Fryer Coconut Shrimp

**Prep Time: 10 minutes  Cook Time: 12 minutes  Servings: 4**

### INGREDIENTS

- 1 pound shrimp raw, large, peeled and deveined with tails attached
- ¼ cup all-purpose flour
- ½ teaspoon salt
- ¼ teaspoon black pepper
- 2 large eggs
- ¾ cup unsweetened shredded coconut
- ¼ cup breadcrumbs
- Cooking spray
- Sweet chili sauce for serving

### DIRECTIONS

1. Preheat the air fryer to 360°F. When heated, spray the basket with cooking spray.
2. Combine the flour, salt and pepper in one shallow bowl. Whisk the eggs in a second shallow bowl. Then combine the shredded coconut and panko breadcrumbs in a third shallow bowl.
3. Dip the shrimp into the flour mixture, shaking off any excess. Then dredge the shrimp into the eggs, and finally into the coconut panko mixture, gently pressing to adhere.
4. Place the coconut shrimp in the air fryer so they are not touching, and spray the top of the shrimp. Cook for 10-12 minutes, flipping halfway through.
5. Garnish with chopped parsley, and serve immediately with sweet chili sauce, if desired.

# Air Fryer Korean BBQ Cauliflower Wings

**Prep Time: 15 minutes** **Cook Time: 15 minutes** **Servings: 4**

## INGREDIENTS

- 1 head cauliflower medium
- 2 cups panko bread crumbs
- 3 eggs large
- Korean BBQ Sauce
- 1/4 cup hoisin sauce
- 1/3 cup honey
- 1 tbsp soy sauce
- 1 tbsp rice vinegar
- 1 tbsp ketchup
- 1 tsp sesame oil
- 1/4 tsp ground ginger
- 2 cloves garlic minced
- 1/4 cup water cold
- 2 tsp corn starch

## DIRECTIONS

1. Preheat air-fryer or convection oven to 400 F
2. Wash and dry a medium head of cauliflower. Cut cauliflower crown bit-size pieces removing any stems.
3. In a small bowl add 3 large eggs beat. In a large bowl add 2 cups of panko bread crumbs. Dip each piece of cauliflower first in the egg mixture and then into the panko bread crumbs. Before adding each piece to the panko bread crumbs be sure to shake off any excess egg. Toss the cauliflower in the panko bread crumbs and then place on a wire rack that will sit on top of the baking sheet. Ensure the cauliflower pieces are not touching or crowded so there is room for air to fully circulate around each piece. Air-fry or bake for 15 minutes. If using a convection oven flip the cauliflower pieces halfway through cooking.
4. Meanwhile in a small pot over medium-high heat add 1/4 cup hoisin sauce, 1/3 cup honey, 1 tbsp soy sauce, 1 tbsp ketchup, 1 tbsp rice vinegar, 1 tsp sesame oil, 1/4 tsp ground ginger and 2 minced garlic cloves. Stir to combine and let come to a small boil.
5. In a small bowl add 1/4 cup of cold water and 2 tsp of cornstarch. Mix well until cornstarch has been fully dissolved. Pour into the BBQ sauce mixture and mix well. Reduce heat to medium and continue to simmer the sauce until it thickens. About 2-3 minutes.
6. Transfer the cooked cauliflower pieces to a large bowl ad add the sauce. Toss until each cauliflower wing is fully coated. Serve immediately.

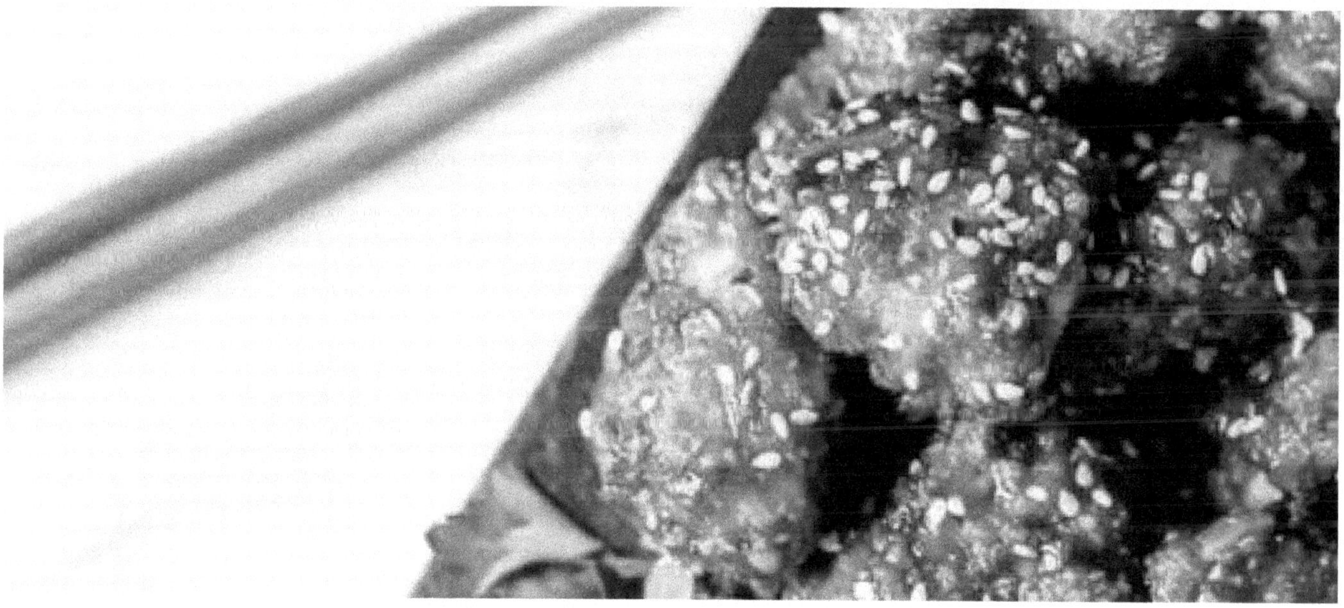

# Creamy Vegan Cauliflower Gnocchi

**Total Time: 25 minutes** **Servings: 2**

## INGREDIENTS

- 1 package store-bought cauliflower gnocchi (I used Trader Joe's)
- 2 tbsp olive oil
- kosher salt and ground black pepper
- 1/2 up diced red onion
- 3 cloves of garlic (minced)
- 1 pint baby bella mushrooms
- 1/3 cup vegetable stock
- 1 tbsp dried basil or oregano
- 1 cup coconut milk (full-fat)
- 1 cup fresh spinach
- 1/2 cup grated parmesan cheese (if not making this fully vegan)
- 1/4 cup fresh chopped parsley

## DIRECTIONS

### PREPARE THE CAULIFLOWER GNOCCHI

1. Now, there are a couple of methods suggested on the package but the preferred way and I agree is to steam it in a pan on the stove then sauté it so the bottoms get nice and crispy brown.
2. To do this you just add the gnocchi (frozen) to a sauté pan on the stovetop with some water, cover and steam it for about 5-6 minutes. You want all of the water to become absorbed. Then just add a little butter or oil to the pan, turn up the heat to medium-high heat and let those little babies get nice and crispy. This takes about 3-4 minutes. Season the gnocchi with salt and pepper and set it aside while you prepare the rest of the ingredients.

### MAKE THE CREAMY VEGGIE-FILLED SAUCE

3. Heat up a skillet to medium heat with 1 tablespoon of olive oil. Once the oil is hot, add in the diced red onion, mushrooms and garlic. Let that cook for 4-5 minutes, stirring occasionally until the mushrooms start to get nice and golden brown.
4. Add in the spinach and cook until wilted, about 1-2 minutes.
5. Pour in the vegetable stock, dried basil or oregano and stir to combine it with the veggies. Season with more salt and pepper. Let that come to a simmer and cook for 2-3 minutes.
6. Next, add in the coconut milk and stir it in with all of those deliciously simmered veggies and let that all cook for 2 more minutes.

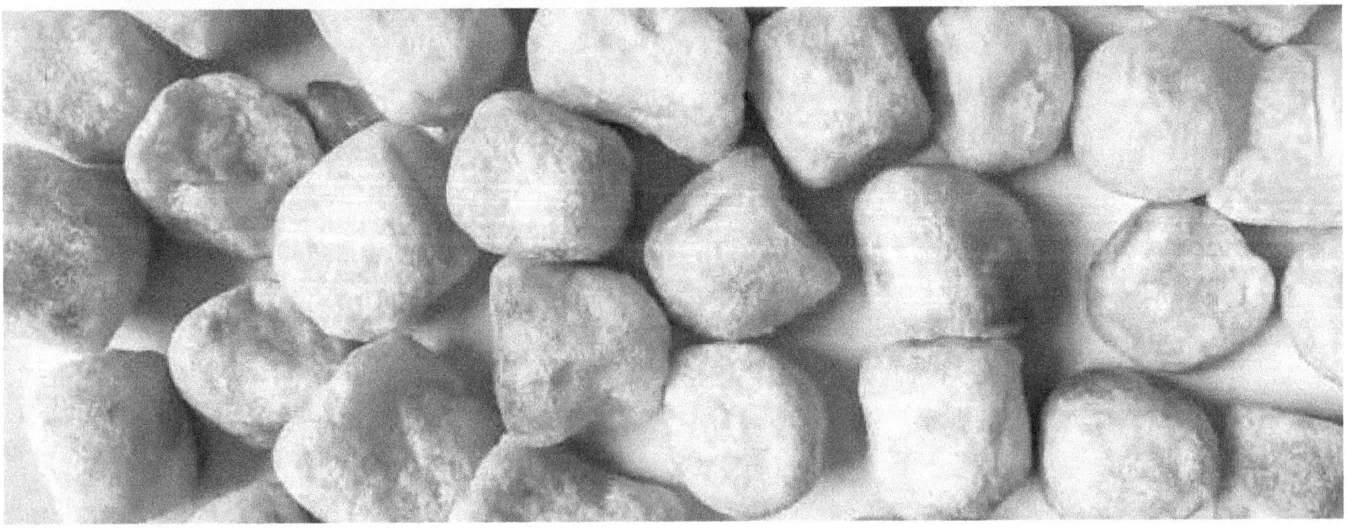

# Air Fryer Glazed Donuts

**Prep Time: 30 minutes** **Cook Time: 4 minutes** **Servings: 12**

## INGREDIENTS

- 1 cup milk lukewarm (about 100°F)°
- 2 1/2 tsp active dry yeast or instant yeast
- 1/4 cup granulated sugar plus 1 tsp
- 1/2 tsp salt
- 1 egg
- 1/4 cup unsalted butter melted
- 3 cups all-purpose flour
- Oil Spray Coconut oil works best
- For the Glaze
- 6 Tbsp unsalted butter
- 2 cups powdered sugar
- 2 tsp vanilla extract
- 4 Tbsp hot water or as needed

## DIRECTIONS

1. In the bowl of a stand mixer fitted with the dough hook, gently stir together lukewarm milk, 1 tsp of sugar, and yeast. Let it sit for 10 minutes until foamy (If nothing happens your milk was too hot or the yeast is too old, so start over).
2. Add sugar, salt, egg, melted butter and 2 cups of flour to the milk mixture. Mix on low speed until combined, then with the mixer running add the remaining cup of flour slowly, until the dough no longer sticks to the bowl. Increase speed to medium-low and knead for 5 minutes, until the dough is elastic and smooth.
3. Place the dough into a greased bowl and cover it with plastic wrap. Let rise in a warm place until doubled. Dough is ready if you make a dent with your finger and the indention remains.
4. Turn the dough out onto a floured surface, punch it down and gently roll out to about 1/2 inch thickness. Cut out 10-12 donuts using a 3-inch round cutter and a 1-inch round cutter to remove center.
5. Transfer donuts and donut holes to lightly floured parchment paper and cover loosely with greased plastic wrap. Let donuts rise until doubled in volume, about 30 minutes. Preheat Air Fryer to 350F.
6. Spray Air Fryer basket with oil spray, carefully transfer donuts to Air Fryer basket in a single layer. Spray donuts with oil spray and cook at 350F until golden brown, about 4 minutes. Repeat with remaining donuts and holes.
7. While the donuts are in the Air Fryer, melt butter in a small saucepan over medium heat. Stir in powdered sugar and vanilla extract until smooth. Remove from heat and stir in hot water one tablespoon at a time until the icing is somewhat thin, but not watery. Set aside.
8. Dip hot donuts and donut holes in the glaze using to forks to submerge them. Place on a wire rack set over a rimmed baking sheet to allow excess glaze to drip off. Let sit until glaze hardens, about 10 minutes.

# Air Fryer Chicken Nuggets

**Prep Time: 10 minutes Cook Time: 8 minutes Servings: 4**

## INGREDIENTS

**cooking/oil spray**

- 2 chicken breasts cut into 1″ to 1.5″ cubes
- 1/3 cup olive oil more if needed
- 1.5 cup panko
- 1/4 cup parmesan
- 2 tsp sweet paprika

## DIRECTIONS

1. Cut up your chicken breasts into 1″ to 1.5″ cubes and set them aside.
2. Set up your station with one bowl holding your olive oil, and the other holding your panko, parmesan, and paprika mix.
3. Spritz the inside of your air fryer lightly with some oil.
4. Dip your chicken cube into the olive oil, then place it into your coating. Make sure your nugget is well coated and place it into the air fryer. Repeat until your air fryer is full. Do not over crowd the air fryer, air fry in batches if needed.
5. Set your air fryer to 400F and cook your homemade chicken nuggets for 8 minutes.
6. Serve with your choice of dip.

◇◇◇◇◇◇◇◇◇◇◇◇◇◇◇◇◇◇◇◇◇◇◇◇◇◇◇◇◇◇◇◇◇◇◇◇◇◇◇◇◇◇

# Air Fryer Baked Apples

**Prep Time: 5 minutes Cook Time: 15 minutes Servings: 2**

## INGREDIENTS

- 2 Apples (I use Pink Lady)
- 1 tsp Butter, melted
- 1/2 tsp Cinnamon

**TOPPING INGREDIENTS**

- 1/3 cup Old Fashioned / Rolled Oats
- 1 tbsp Butter, melted
- 1 tbsp Maple Syrup (or honey or rice malt syrup)
- 1 tsp Wholemeal / Whole Wheat Flour, (can sub for almond meal or all purpose flour / plain flour)
- 1/2 tsp Cinnamon

## DIRECTIONS

1. Cut apples in half through the stem and use a knife or a spoon to remove the core, stem and seeds. Brush a tsp of butter evenly over the cut sides of the apples, then sprinkle over 1/2 tsp of cinnamon.
2. Mix topping ingredients together in a small bowl, then spoon on top of the apple halves evenly.
3. Place the apple halves carefully into the air fryer basket, then cook on 180C / 350F for 15 minutes or until softened.
4. Serve warm with ice cream or cream if desired.

# Air Fryer Copycat Taco Crunchwrap

**Prep Time: 5 minutes Cook Time: 5 minutes Servings: 1**

## INGREDIENTS

- 1 large burrito (10 inch) size tortilla
- 2 tbsp fat free refried beans
- 1/4 cup extra lean ground beef seasoned with taco seasoning
- 2 tbsp reduced fat shredded cheese
- 2 tbsp nacho cheese dip i use the fritos brand cheddar or jalapeno cheese dip, but you can find multiple different brands in the chip aisle! Rico's nacho cheese is also delicious.
- 1 tbsp non fat greek yogurt I prefer Fage. You also can use sour cream.
- 8 bite size tortilla chips I use the Tostitos brand, but any kind of chip will do
- 2 tbsp finely chopped onions and lettuce
- 1 tbsp favorite salsa or a couple finely chopped cherry tomatos work too!
- cooking spray (i prefer to use Avocado oil cooking spray)

## DIRECTIONS

1. Make a cut into the middle of the tortilla and only go to the middle. (Pictures in blog post will describe this best, once you see it, you won't forget it!)
2. Look at the tortilla and divide the ingredients into four quadrants. On the left half spread the cheese dip then pile on the broken tortilla chips in one quadrant and ground beef in the other quadrant. On the remaining spread nonfat greek yogurt in one of the quadrants then add lettuce, onion, salsa (or tomatoes). In the last quadrant spread the refriend beans then add the shredded cheese on top.
3. Fold: First fold the bottom left quadrant up over the upper left quadrant then fold that over onto the upper right quadrant then fold all of those back down onto the bottom right quadrant. The end of result will look like a triangle.
4. I know this might not make sense in written form so if you haven't seen the tortilla folding method yet please check out the step by step photos on my blog post above. It will make much better sense. Once you do it once you won't forget it!
5. You don't have to heat this up, but I would especially if your filling ingredients aren't warmed up. I do prefer it warmed up.
6. Air Fryer: Spray each side lightly with a little bit of cooking spray then place in the air fryer and heat until lightly golden brown at 350 degrees for about 5-6 minutes.
7. Skillet: Heat skillet over medium heat and spray each side of the wrap lightly with cooking spray. Heat each side for 2-3 minutes or until lightly golden brown.

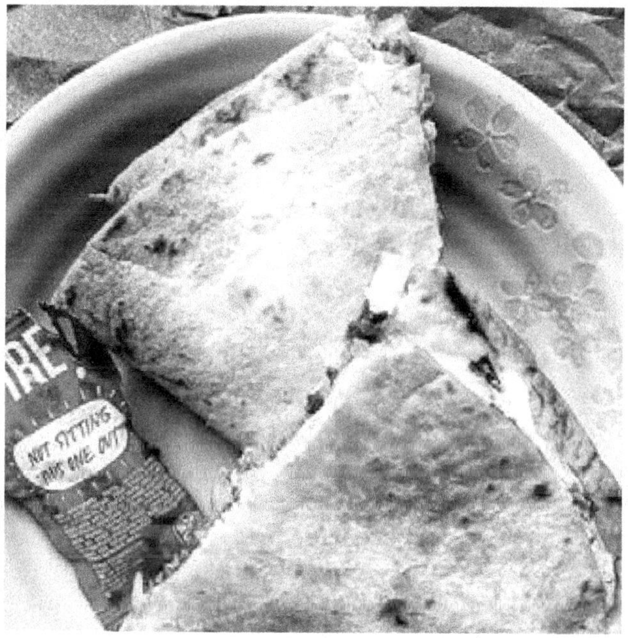

# Air Fryer Sweet Potato Chips

**Prep Time: 5 minutes  Cook Time: 15 minutes  Servings: 2**

### INGREDIENTS

- 1 large sweet potato, or yam
- 1 tablespoon olive oil
- 1 ½ teaspoons kosher salt
- ½ teaspoon pepper
- 1 teaspoon dried thyme

### DIRECTIONS

1. Preheat the air fryer to 350°F (180°C).
2. Cut the sweet potato into ⅛-¼-inch (3- to 6-mm) slices. In a medium bowl, toss the sweet potato slices with the olive oil until well coated. Add the salt, pepper, and thyme and toss to coat.
3. Working in batches, add the sweet potato chips to the air fryer in a single layer and "fry" for 14 minutes, until golden brown and lightly crispy.
4. Enjoy!

◊◊◊◊◊◊◊◊◊◊◊◊◊◊◊◊◊◊◊◊◊◊◊◊◊◊◊◊◊◊◊◊◊◊◊◊◊◊

# Crispy Air Fryer Fish Cakes

**Prep Time: 15 minutes  Cook Time: 10 minutes  Servings: 4**

### INGREDIENTS

- 12 ounces cod fillets, or any other white fish, coarsely chopped
- 2/3 cup pork rind panko crumbs, you can also use regular breadcrumbs
- 2 tablespoons finely chopped fresh cilantro
- 2 tablespoons sweet chili sauce
- 2 tablespoons mayonnaise
- 1 egg
- ¼ teaspoon salt, or to taste
- ¼ teaspoon fresh ground black pepper, or to taste
- Lime wedges, for serving

### DIRECTIONS

1. Preheat air fryer to 400˚F.
2. Grease the basket of the air fryer with non-aerosol cooking spray, or line it with parchment paper.
3. Transfer the chopped fish to a food processor and process until crumbly. (see notes below)
4. In a bowl combine the crumbled fish, pork rind crumbs, cilantro, chili sauce, mayo, egg, salt, and pepper; stir until well incorporated.
5. Shape the mixture into four patties.
6. Place the patties in the air fryer basket and coat them with cooking spray.
7. Cook for 5 minutes; flip over the fish cakes, spray with cooking spray, and continue to cook for 4 to 5 more minutes, or until golden brown and crispy.
8. Remove from air fryer basket.
9. Serve fish cakes with lime wedges.

# Air Fryer Cheeseburger Sliders

**Prep Time: 10 minutes** **Cook Time: 15 minutes** **Servings: 9**

## INGREDIENTS

- 1 pound ground beef, crumbled
- ½ teaspoon garlic salt
- ½ teaspoon onion flakes
- ½ teaspoon ground black pepper
- 2 oz. cream cheese, cut into small cubes
- 4 tablespoons barbecue sauce
- 1 ½ cups grated cheddar-jack cheese or Mexican cheese blend
- 1 pkg. Hawaiian rolls (may not use all)
- ¼ cup salted butter, melted
- 1-2 teaspoons sesame seeds
- Sliced dill pickles (for garnish)

## DIRECTIONS

1. Crumble ground beef into a small pan or baking dish that will fit into the air fryer.
2. Add garlic salt, onion flakes, and black pepper and mix well with your fingertips to combine.
3. Slice the sheet of rolls in half and set the top section aside—place bottoms of rolls into the air fryer basket on top of the aluminum foil.
4. Cook ground beef in the air fryer at 400°F for 5 minutes. Stir and continue cooking until ground beef has fully browned. (This took 10 minutes in my 1800 W air fryer.)
5. Remove the pan from the air fryer basket and drain any excess oil/liquid.
6. Add cubed cream cheese and barbecue sauce to the ground beef and mix well with a spatula to fully combine. Set aside.
7. Keeping the Hawaiian rolls attached, measure to determine how many will fit into the basket of your air fryer at once. Tear off any rolls that won't fit and use in a second batch or set aside for another use. (My air fryer basket held a neat square of 9 rolls.)
8. Line the basket of the air fryer with aluminum foil.
9. Slice the sheet of rolls in half and set the top section aside—place bottoms of rolls into the air fryer basket on top of the aluminum foil.
10. Cover the roll bottoms with about 1 cup of cheese. (You can also use cheese slices, but freshly grated cheese seems to melt faster.)
11. Pile ground beef mixture over the cheese and pat it into an even layer.
12. Sprinkle additional cheese over the ground beef, if desired.
13. Place the tops of the rolls over the prepared sliders.
14. Brush melted butter over the top of the sliders using a pastry brush. Don't be afraid to use all of the butter. Extra that runs off the sides will be caught by the aluminum foil, helping the butter soak in and crisp up the rolls' bottoms.
15. Sprinkle with sesame seeds, if desired.
16. Place the basket in the air fryer and cook for 4-5 minutes (at 400 degrees F, air fryer setting) or until the cheese has melted and the tops are browned, and the sliders are heated through. If needed, cover with aluminum foil at the end of the cooking time to prevent the tops from getting overly browned while the cheese is still melting.
17. Plate, serve, and enjoy!

# Air Fryer BBQ Ribs

**Prep Time: 2 minutes    Cook Time: 28 minutes    Servings: 4**

## INGREDIENTS

**Ribs and Dry Rub:**

- 3 pounds baby back pork ribs (1 rack)
- 3 teaspoons garlic powder
- 2 teaspoons paprika
- 1 teaspoon salt
- 1/2 teaspoon black pepper
- 1/2 teaspoon cuminutes
- Sweet and Sticky BBQ Sauce
- 1/2 cup ketchup
- 2 tablespoons brown sugar
- 1 tablespoon apple cider vinegar
- 1 tablespoon olive oil
- 1/2 teaspoon ground cuminutes
- salt and pepper to taste

## DIRECTIONS

1. Remove the membrane: Peel off the silverskin from the back of the ribs.
2. Cut the rack of pork ribs into 2-3 sections so that it can fit into your air fryer basket.
3. Make the spice rub: In a small bowl, mix garlic powder, paprika, salt, pepper and cumin.
4. Season the baby back ribs: Pat the ribs dry and rub the ribs on all sides with the spice rub.
5. Cook the ribs in the air fryer: Preheat the air fryer to 375°F/190°C for a few minutes. Once hot, place the ribs into the basket with the meat side down and cook for 15 minutes. (It's important to let the air fryer to heat up first to avoid the ribs from sticking to the basket.)
6. Flip the ribs using kitchen tongs, and cook for 10 more minutes at 375°F/190°C.
7. Make the BBQ sauce: While the ribs are cooking, you can add bbq sauce ingredients in a saucepan. Heat over medium-low heat until the sugar and salt are completely dissolved.
8. Brush with BBQ sauce: Remove the basket from the air fryer and brush generously with barbecue sauce on all sides.
9. Place the basket back in the air fryer and cook for 3-5 more minutes at 400°F/200°C, or until the sauce has set and darkened slightly. (It may take more or less time based on the thickness or your ribs)
10. Remove the ribs from the basket and let them rest for 5 minutes so that the juices can redistribute through the meat. Feel free to brush with more barbeque sauce if you like.

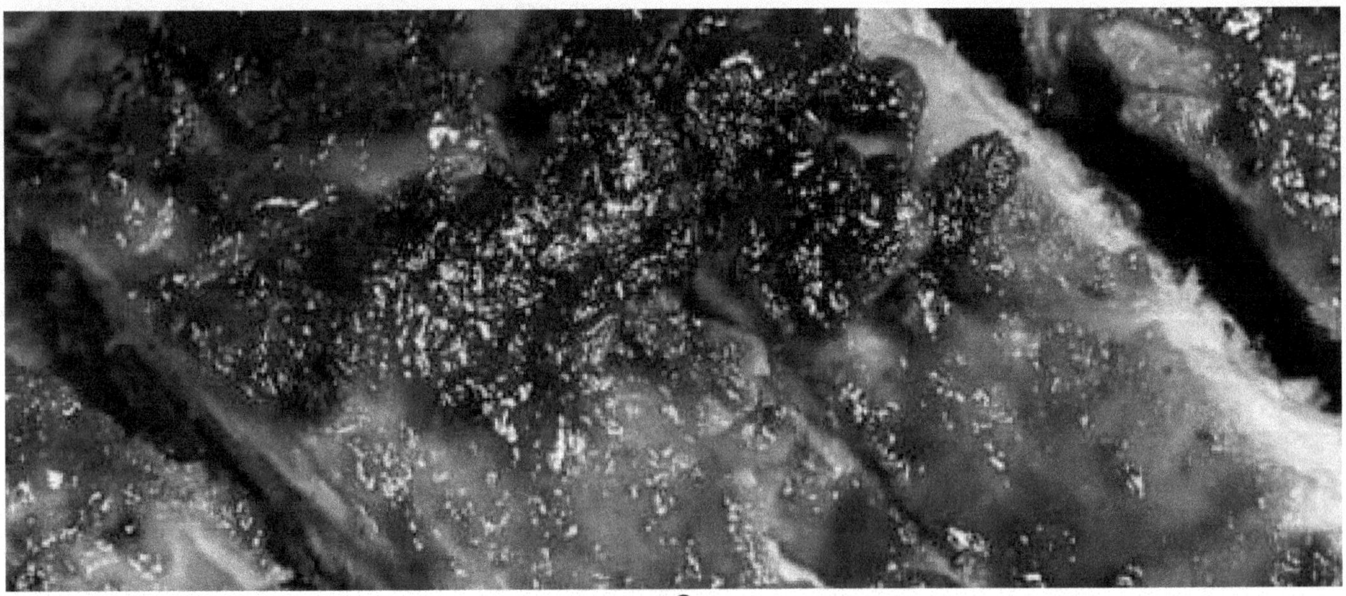

# Air Fryer Meatballs

**Prep Time: 5 minutes Cook Time: 20 minutes Servings: 4**

**INGREDIENTS**

- 1 lb ground beef
- 1/2 cup dried bread crumbs
- 1/2 cup grated Parmesan cheese
- 1/4 cup milk
- 2 cloves garlic minced
- 1/2 tsp Italian seasoning
- 3/4 tsp salt
- 1/4 tsp pepper

**DIRECTIONS**

1. Combine all ingredients in a bowl, then roll into 1 1/2 inch meatballs.
2. Put the meatballs into an air fryer basket in a single layer, without them touching.
3. Air fry the meatballs at 375F for 15 minutes.

# Crispy Breaded Air Fryer Chicken Breast

**Prep Time: 5 minutes Cook Time: 15 minutes Servings: 4**

**INGREDIENTS**

- 1 Lb Chicken breast
- 2 tsp Olive oil
- Salt
- 1/2 Cup Panko (GF if needed)
- 2 tsp Seasoning salt
- 2 tsp Paprika
- 2 tsp Ground mustard powder
- 2 tsp Garlic powder
- 2 tsp Onion powder

**DIRECTIONS**

1. Preheat your air fryer to 400 degrees.
2. Place the chicken breast between two layers of parchment paper. Use a rolling pin or meat mallet to gentle press the chicken so it's an even width throughout. Dry the chicken breasts off with paper towel.
3. Pour the oil onto the chicken (I do this right on the parchment) and rub all over, coating it equally. Sprinkle with a pinch of salt.
4. Combine the rest of the ingredients in a small bowl, shaking together. Pour onto a large rimmed plate.
5. Cover each of the chicken breasts well with the panko mixture, and then place onto the mesh basket of your air fryer, making sure to leave room between the breasts - they would not be touching.
6. Spray the tops of the chicken with cooking spray and cook 8 minutes. Gently flip and cook another 6-8 minutes until the chicken is crispy and golden and an instant read thermometer reads 165 degrees Fahrenheit inserted into the chicken
7. DEVOUR! (Great with ketchup! ?

# Air Fryer Chicken Quesadilla

**Prep Time: 3 minutes  Cook Time: 10 minutes  Servings: 4**

### INGREDIENTS

- Air Fryer Chicken Quesadilla Ingredients:
- 2 corn tortillas gluten-free
- 3 tablespoons guacamole
- 1/3 cup cheddar cheese grated
- 1/2 cup (about 100g) cooked chicken breast cubed

### DIRECTIONS

1. Air Fryer Chicken Quesadilla Recipe Directions
2. Preheat air fryer to 325 F / 170 C.
3. Lightly spray the air fryer basket with olive oil.
4. Set the first tortilla inside the basket. Then spread on the guacamole, add the cheese and chicken and then top with the second tortilla.
5. Use a toothpick to hold the top tortilla in place during cooking.
6. Cook for 6-10 minutes (depending on how crispy you like them), carefully flipping the quesadilla over halfway through.
7. Remove from the air fryer, cut and serve.

◇◇◇◇◇◇◇◇◇◇◇◇◇◇◇◇◇◇◇◇◇◇◇◇◇◇◇◇◇◇◇◇◇◇◇◇◇◇◇◇

# Air Fryer Twice Baked Potatoes

**Prep Time: 5 minutes  Cook Time: 10 minutes  Servings: 4**

### INGREDIENTS

- 2 cooked baked potatoes
- 2 Tablespoon sour cream
- 1/2 cup cheddar cheese
- 1 Tablespoon butter
- 2 slices bacon, cooked

### DIRECTIONS

1. Cut the baked potatoes in half and scoop out the insides into a bowl.
2. Add the sour cream, 1/4 cup of cheddar cheese and the butter to the bowl with the potatoes.
3. Mash the potatoes and other ingredients together with a potato masher until they have reached your desired consistency.
4. Spoon the filling back into the potato shells, mounding it to fit as necessary.
5. Refrigerate until ready to serve.
6. When you are ready to bake the potatoes put them in an air fryer basket. Cook at 400 F for 8 minutes.
7. Top the potatoes with the remaining 1/4 cup of cheddar cheese and bacon bits. Be careful not to touch the hot sides of the air fryer basket while you do this.
8. Return the potatoes to the air fryer and cook for 2 more minutes at 400 F to melt the cheese and crisp the bacon.

# Air Fryer Buffalo Cauliflower Bites

**Prep Time: 10 minutes Cook Time: 15 minutes Servings: 4**

## INGREDIENTS

- 1 head cauliflower, cut into florets (you'll need about 4 to 5 cups)
- 2 tablespoons butter, melted
- 1 tablespoon olive oil
- 1/2 cup Frank's Red Hot Sauce
- 1/2 cup almond flour
- 3 tablespoons dried parsley
- 1/2 tablespoon garlic powder
- 1 teaspoon Lawry's Seasoning Salt

## DIRECTIONS

1. Place cauliflower florets in a large mixing bowl and set aside.
2. Melt butter; stir in olive oil and hot sauce until thoroughly combined.
3. Pour the hot sauce mixture over the cauliflower; mix around until all cauliflower florets are coated.
4. In a separate bowl whisk together almond flour, dried parsley, garlic powder, and seasoning salt.
5. Sprinkle about a handful at a time of almond flour mixture over the cauliflower; gently mix until everything is coated.
6. Transfer half of the prepared cauliflower to the air fryer.
7. Air fry at 350°F for 15 minutes, shaking a couple times during the cooking process. Cauliflower is done when the florets are a bit browned, but not mushy.
8. Remove cauliflower from the Air Fryer; set aside and keep covered.
9. Repeat the same process with the remaining cauliflower florets.
10. Serve with celery sticks and your favorite bleu cheese dressing.

# Air Fryer Pork Chops

**Prep Time: 5 minutes Cook Time: 9 minutes Servings: 4**

## INGREDIENTS

- 4 Boneless pork chops approximately 1 inch thick
- 1 tablespoon Olive oil
- 2 teaspoon Garlic powder
- 2 teaspoon Onion powder
- 2 teaspoon Paprika
- 1 teaspoon Salt
- 1/2 teaspoon Pepper

## DIRECTIONS

1. In a small bowl combine garlic powder, onion powder, salt, and paprika.
2. Brush the pork chops with a light coating of olive oil and then rub your spice mix into them.
3. Working in batches place your pork chops in the airy fryer basket. Do not stack the pork chops, place them side-by-side.
4. Set the temperature to 375 degrees F and the timer to 9 minutes. Start cooking the pork chops.
5. Halfway through stop the timer and remove the basket, flipping the pork chops over. Replace the basket and start timer.
6. When done check the internal temperature to ensure that it is 145 degrees F and then remove the pork chops from the air fryer and let rest for 3 minutes before serving.

# Air Fryer Egg Rolls

**Cook Time: 15 minutes  Prep Time: 15 minutes  Air Frying: 16 minutes  Servings: 12**

## INGREDIENTS

- 1/2 pound ground pork
- 1/2 onion
- 1/2 bag coleslaw mix
- 4 ounces mushrooms
- 1 stalk celery
- 1/2 teaspoon salt
- egg roll wrappers

## DIRECTIONS

1. Heat a skillet over medium heat.
2. Add the ground pork and onion and cook until pork is no longer pink.
3. Add the mushrooms, celery, coleslaw mixture and salt to the skillet. Cook for 5 minutes to soften the vegetables.
4. Put the wrapper on a cutting board. Add 1/3 cup of filling mixture to the top corner of the egg roll wrapper. Fold the top down over the filling. Then roll the wrapper up, tucking the sides in as you go. When you get to the bottom use your fingers to moisten the edges of the wrapper and seal it in place.
5. Continue to roll the egg rolls until the filling is gone.
6. Spray the egg rolls lightly with cooking spray if desired. This will ensure even browning of the egg rolls.
7. Cook the egg rolls at 400F for 6-8 minutes, flipping once with tongs half way through.

◇◇◇◇◇◇◇◇◇◇◇◇◇◇◇◇◇◇◇◇◇◇◇◇◇◇◇◇◇◇◇◇◇◇◇◇◇

# Air Fryer Pasta Chips

**Prep Time: 15 minutes  Cook Time: 10 minutes  Servings: 1**

## INGREDIENTS

- 1 pound bowtie pasta
- 3 tablespoons olive oil
- 1/4 cup grated Parmesan cheese
- 1 teaspoon Italian seasoning
- 1 teaspoon garlic powder
- 1 teaspoon crushed red pepper

## DIRECTIONS

1. Bring a large pot of salted water to a boil.
2. Add pasta and cook according to box directions until al dente.
3. Drain pasta and add to a large mixing bowl.
4. Add olive to pasta and toss.
5. Add in grated Parmesan cheese, Italian seasoning, garlic powder, and crushed red pepper.
6. Toss to combine.
7. Preheat air fryer to 400 degrees F.
8. Add pasta to preheated air fryer, covering the bottom of the basket and not overlapping in the basket.
9. Cook for 4 minutes on 400 degrees F.
10. Toss and cook for another 4-5 minutes at 400 degrees F. until you have reached your desired crispness.
11. Continue until all pasta chips have been made.
12. Serve with marinara sauce for dipping.

# Air Fryer Tortilla Chips

**Prep Time: 5 minutes** **Cook Time: 5 minutes** **Servings: 2**

**INGREDIENTS**

- 12 corn tortillas
- 1 tablespoon olive oil
- 2 teaspoons kosher salt
- 1 tablespoon McCormick® TASTY Jazzy Spice Blend
- guacamole, for serving

**DIRECTIONS**

1. Preheat the air fryer to 350°F (180°C).
2. Lightly brush the tortillas with olive oil on both sides.
3. Sprinkle the tortillas with the salt and Tasty Jazzy Spice Blend on both sides.
4. Cut each tortilla into 6 wedges.
5. Working in batches, add the tortilla wedges to the air fryer in a single layer and "fry" for about 5 minutes, or until golden brown and crispy.
6. Serve with guacamole.
7. Enjoy!

# Crispy Air Fryer Fish Fillets

**Prep Time**: **5 minutes** **Cook Time**: **15 minutes** **Servings**: **8**

**INGREDIENTS**

- 8 (28oz, 800g) fish fillets
- 1 tablespoon olive oil or vegetable oil
- 1 cup (50g) dry bread crumbs If following a gluten-free diet, use gluten-free breadcrumbs.
- ½ teaspoon paprika
- ¼ teaspoon chili powder
- ¼ teaspoon ground black pepper
- ¼ teaspoon garlic powder or granules
- ¼ teaspoon onion powder
- ½ teaspoon salt

**For Serving:**

- tartar sauce
- lemon wedges

**DIRECTIONS**

1. If using frozen fish fillets, defrost them. Drizzle with olive oil, and make sure that the fish is well coated with oil.
2. In a shallow dish, mix the bread crumbs with paprika, chili powder, black pepper, garlic powder, onion powder and salt.
3. Coat each fish fillet in bread crumbs, and transfer to your air fryer basket.
4. Cook in the air fryer at 390°F (200°C) for 12-15 minutes. After the first 8-10 minutes, open the air fryer and flip the fish fillets on the other side then continue cooking.

## Air Fryer Homemade Croutons

**Prep Time: 5 minutes Cook Time: 12 minutes Servings: 6**

### INGREDIENTS

- 3-4 Cups Stale Bread – cubed (1/2 large loaf or 1 small loaf)
- 2-3 Tablespoons Olive Oil
- Salt
- Dried Italian Seasoning

### DIRECTIONS

1. Cut stale bread loaf into approximately 1 inch cubes. Transfer bread cubes to large bowl.
2. Drizzle olive oil over bread. Sprinkle with salt and seasoning.
3. Using your hands, gently toss bread cubes until evenly coated.
4. Transfer bread to air fryer basket that has been sprayed with nonstick.
5. Air fry croutons at 350°F for 10-12 minutes or until crisp golden brown. Toss once during cook time.

◇◇◇◇◇◇◇◇◇◇◇◇◇◇◇◇◇◇◇◇◇◇◇◇◇◇◇◇◇◇◇◇◇◇◇◇◇◇◇◇◇◇◇◇◇◇◇◇◇◇

## Air Fryer Peanut Butter Cookies

**Prep Time: 10 minutes Cook Time: 7 minutes Servings: 9**

### INGREDIENTS

- 1 3/4 cups all purpose flour regular or gluten free
- 3/4 teaspoon baking soda
- 1/2 teaspoon salt
- 1/2 cup butter softened to room temperature
- 1/2 cup peanut butter smooth
- 1/2 cup brown sugar
- 1/2 cup sugar
- egg
- 2 tablespoons milk dairy or non-dairy

### DIRECTIONS

1. In a medium sized bowl, mix together all purpose flour and baking soda. Set aside.
2. In another bowl, mix together softened butter and peanut butter. It may help to use an electric mixer. Add sugars and mix until well combined.
3. Next, add the egg and milk. Mix well to combine.
4. Slowly add the flour mixture in small increments. Mix until just combined. Do not overmix.
5. Roll about a tablespoon of cookie dough into a ball. Use a fork to flatten the cookie. Place cookies into air fryer basket or onto air fryer tray.
6. Air fry the cookies for 6 to 7 minutes at 350 degrees F or 180 degrees C.
7. Remove cookies from air fryer. Cookies should rest until completely cool to strengthen. Enjoy!

# Honey Lime Air Fryer Shrimp

**Prep Time: 5 minutes Cook Time: 5 minutes Servings: 4**

**INGREDIENTS**

- 1 lb large shrimp raw; remove shell and tail if desired; note 1
- 1 1/2 tablespoons olive oil
- 1 1/2 tablespoons lime juice note 2
- 1 1/2 tablespoons honey note 3
- 2 cloves garlic minced
- 1/8 teaspoon salt
- To garnish
- lime wedges
- cilantro

**DIRECTIONS**

1. Marinade - In a large bowl, stir together the olive oil, lime juice, honey, garlic and salt. Add the shrimp and marinate for 20-30 minutes.
2. Cook - Heat the air fryer to 390°F/200°C.Shake excess marinade off the shrimp and put the whole batch in the air fryer.
3. Cook for 2 minutes, give the basket a good shake, and return to the air fryer. Cook for another 2-3 minutes, or until shrimp are pink and cooked through.
4. Serve - with lime wedges and cilantro.

◇◇◇◇◇◇◇◇◇◇◇◇◇◇◇◇◇◇◇◇◇◇◇◇◇◇◇◇◇◇◇◇◇◇◇◇◇◇

# Air Fryer Cinnamon Rolls

**Prep Time: 8 minutes Cook Time: 7 minutes Servings: 8**

**INGREDIENTS**

**Cinnamon rolls:**

- 1 tablespoon Ground Cinnamon
- ¾ stick Unsalted Butter , softened (80 grams)
- 6 tablespoons Brown Sugar
- 1 Sheet Puff Pastry , thawed (see note 1)
- Icing:
- ½ cup Powdered Sugar
- 1 tablespoon Milk
- 2 teaspoons Fresh Lemon Juice

**DIRECTIONS**

1. In a small bowl, combine cinnamon, softened butter and sugar. Mix well.
2. Preheat the air fryer to 400° Fahrenheit (200° Celsius) for 4 minutes.
3. Gently roll out (or unroll, if using ready-rolled pastry) the pastry and spread the cinnamon mixture across the whole sheet – in a thin layer.
4. Roll it very gently and loosely (without applying any pressure), starting from the shorter end. This way you will achieve a good amount of swirls. If you start from the wider end, you might not have enough swirls and the cinnamon rolls will kind of unroll when cooking so they will not look so pretty. If you don't mind this, then go ahead and roll them from the wider end.
5. With a serrated knife or flavor-free dental floss, cut the pastry into about 1-inch (2.5 centimeters) pieces.
6. Transfer them to a preheated air fryer and cook at 400° Fahrenheit (200° Celsius) for 7 minutes or until the rolls are puffed and golden brown (see note 6).
7. When ready, take them out, let them cool slightly before topping them with icing made by combining powdered sugar, milk and lemon juice.
8. Enjoy while warm!

# Air Fryer Stuffed Mushrooms

**Prep Time**: **10 minutes** **Cook Time**: **18 minutes** **Servings**: **16**

## INGREDIENTS

- 16 medium mushrooms
- 8 ounces cream cheese softened
- 2 tablespoons bacon crumbled, about 3 slices
- 1/3 cup cheddar cheese shredded, divided
- 2 tablespoons parmesan cheese grated
- ¼ teaspoon garlic powder
- ¼ teaspoon kosher salt or to taste
- ⅛ teaspoon smoked paprika
- 1 green onion thinly sliced

## DIRECTIONS

1. Quickly rinse and dry mushrooms.
2. Remove the stem from the mushroom caps (and scoop out the center using a small spoon if desired).
3. Beat softened cream cheese with a mixer on medium until smooth and fluffy.
4. Add bacon, 3 tablespoons cheddar cheese, parmesan cheese, seasonings, and green onion.
5. Stuff the mixture into the mushroom caps.
6. Preheat air fryer to 400°F. Add mushrooms, reduce heat to 350°F. Cook mushrooms 6 minutes.
7. Open the air fryer and top mushrooms with remaining cheddar. Cook 2 minutes longer.
8. Cool 5 minutes before serving.

◇◇◇◇◇◇◇◇◇◇◇◇◇◇◇◇◇◇◇◇◇◇◇◇◇◇◇◇◇◇◇◇◇◇◇◇◇◇◇◇◇

# Air Fryer Steak

**Prep Time**: **10 minutes** **Cook Time**: **15 minutes** **Servings**: **2**

## INGREDIENTS

- 2 strip loin steaks (1.25" thick; or use any steaks of your choosing)
- 2 tsp salt (plus more to taste)
- 2 tsp black pepper (plus more to taste)
- 2 Tbsp butter (melted)

## DIRECTIONS

1. Sprinkle the steaks with salt and pepper, place on a plate and refrigerate for 2-3 days, uncovered. Flip every 12 hours or so, blotting the juices with a paper towel.
2. This step is recommended for superior tenderness and enhanced flavor, but you can skip it if pressed for time.
3. Remove the steaks from the fridge 45-60 minutes before cooking and let them sit at room temperature.
4. Brush the steaks with melted butter on both sides, place on the rack of your air fryer. Cook at 410F for 15 minutes, without pre-heating, for medium doneness.
5. Cook for about 1 to 2 minutes less for medium rare and rare respectively, and 1-2 minutes more for medium-well and well done respectively. The times will need to be adjusted further if air frying steaks thicker or thinner than 1.25" thick.
6. These cooking times are approximate, so use an instant read thermometer in conjunction with the table in the Notes section.
7. Remove steaks from the air fryer, wrap in foil or wax paper, and let rest for 10 minutes, then serve. Try serving with compound butter, it will add a ton of flavor.

# Air Fryer Mac 'n' Cheese

**Prep Time: 10 minutes** **Cook Time: 45 minutes** **Servings: 4-6**

## INGREDIENTS

- ½ pound dry uncooked pasta (we used elbow macaroni)
- 2 cups whole milk
- 1 cup chicken stock
- 4 tablespoons butter
- 4 tablespoons cream cheese
- 8-ounce package sharp cheddar cheese, shredded
- 1 cup shredded mozzarella cheese
- ¼ teaspoon kosher salt
- ¼ teaspoon white pepper
- 1 teaspoon dry mustard
- Pinch Cayenne pepper
- Few grinds fresh nutmeg

## DIRECTIONS

1. Preheat air fryer on 400 degrees F. for 10 minutes.
2. Rinse pasta under hot tap water for two minutes and drain.
3. Place milk, chicken stock, butter and cream cheese in a glass 4-cup or larger measuring cup and microwave until hot, and the butter melted, about 3-4 minutes. (This just needs to be hot enough to melt the butter and cream cheese, not boiling hot)
4. Mix drained pasta, hot liquid, cheddar, mozzarella, salt, pepper, mustard, cayenne and nutmeg in a large bowl then pour into the Air Fryer handled pan.
5. Spray a round parchment circle with pan spray and place sprayed side down over the macaroni mixture, pressing down to touch the mixture. Cover the top with foil and set into the heated air fryer and cook for 45 minutes.
6. Note: Air fryer wattages vary so check at 35 minutes and cook the additional 5-10 minutes as needed. Our air fryer is an 1800-watt air fryer and our macaroni and cheese took exactly 45 minutes.
7. Remove foil and parchment, stir and serve.

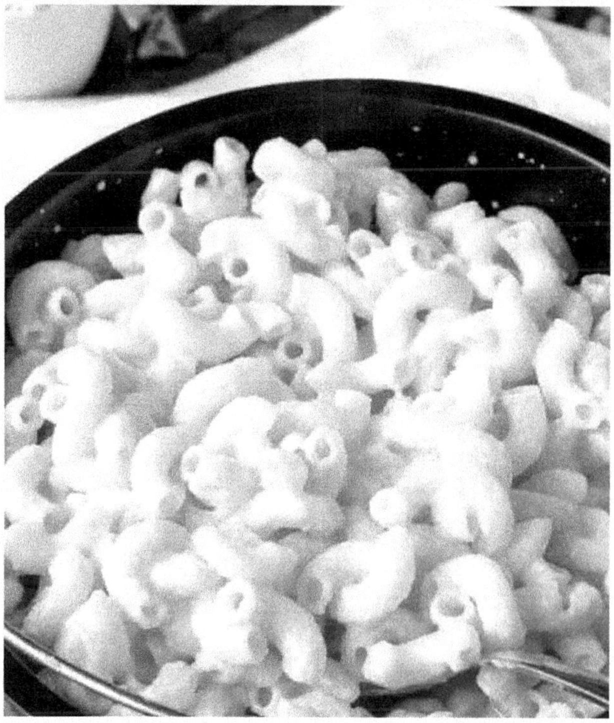

# Air Fryer Nashville Hot Cauliflower Bites

**Prep Time: 30 minutes** **Cook Time: 15 minutes** **Servings: 4**

## INGREDIENTS

**SPICE MIX**

- 1 tablespoon paprika
- 2 teaspoons cayenne
- 2 teaspoons garlic powder
- 2 teaspoons mustard powder
- 2 teaspoons freshly ground black pepper
- 2 teaspoons onion powder

**CAULIFLOWER**

- 1 lb cauliflower florets(150 g)
- 1 teaspoon kosher salt

**BATTER**

- 1 cup buttermilk(240 mL)
- ½ cup all purpose flour(60 g)
- 1 tablespoon louisiana hot sauce
- 1 cup panko breadcrumbs(115 g)
- SPICY OIL
- 1 teaspoon light brown sugar
- 1/3 cup canola oil(80 mL)
- nonstick cooking spray
- FOR SERVING
- white bread
- dill pickle chip

## DIRECTIONS

1. Make the spice mix: In a small bowl, whisk together the paprika, cayenne, garlic powder, mustard powder, black pepper, and onion powder.
2. Add the cauliflower florets to a large bowl and sprinkle with the salt and 2 tablespoons of the spice mix, tossing to coat the cauliflower completely. Cover with plastic wrap and refrigerate for 30 minutes.
3. Preheat the air fryer to 350°F (180°C). Line a baking sheet with foil and place a wire rack on top.
4. Make the batter: In a large bowl, whisk together the buttermilk, flour, and hot sauce until smooth.
5. Add a cauliflower floret to the batter and toss to coat completely.
6. Shake off any excess batter and dip the cauliflower into the panko bread crumbs tossing to coat completely.
7. Spray the air fryer basket with nonstick spray. Add the cauliflower in a single layer, working in batches if necessary. Fry until golden and crispy, about 15 minutes.
8. Make the spicy oil: In a small saucepan, combine 1 tablespoon of the spice mix, the sugar, and canola oil. Cook over medium heat, stirring, for about 2 minutes, until the sugar dissolves.
9. Drizzle the crispy cauliflower with the spicy oil and sprinkle with the remaining spice mix.
10. Serve with white bread and dill pickle chips.
11. Enjoy!

# Air Fryer Chili Garlic Tofu

**Prep Time: 10 minutes  Cook Time: 15 minutes  Servings: 5**

## INGREDIENTS

- 1 package super firm tofu
- 1/2 cup cornstarch, arrowroot, or tapioca
- 1 tablespoon olive oil
- 1/4 cup low-sodium soy sauce
- 2 tablespoons chili garlic sauce
- 1 tablespoon rice vinegar
- 1 1/2 tablespoons swerve or brown sugar
- 2 garlic cloves, minced
- 1 teaspoon grated fresh ginger
- 1 teaspoon sesame oil
- 1/2 teaspoon toasted sesame seeds
- 2 green onions, sliced

## DIRECTIONS

1. Wrap tofu in multiple layers of paper towels. Place a cast iron pan or something heavy on top. Let sit for 30 minutes. Or you can use a tofu press.
2. Cut tofu into cubes.
3. Place cornstarch in a large zip top bag. Shake to coat. Remove tofu pieces, shaking off excess and place in a medium bowl. Drizzle with 1 tablespoon olive oil and gently toss.
4. Place half the tofu pieces in the Air Fryer basket. Set to 370 for 15 minutes. Halfway through open. If they still look powdery, spray them with a little olive oil.
5. Check after about 12 minutes. The cooking time is just an estimate and can vary based on Air Fryer model and size of cubes and brand of tofu.
6. Remove tofu from Air Fryer and set aside. Repeat with remaining tofu.
7. In a nonstick skillet, combine soy sauce, chili garlic sauce, vinegar, sverve, garlic, and ginger. Bring to a boil and simmer for 1 minute.
8. Add sesame oil and tofu and cook and stir for 1 minute.
9. Sprinkle with sesame seeds and green onions.

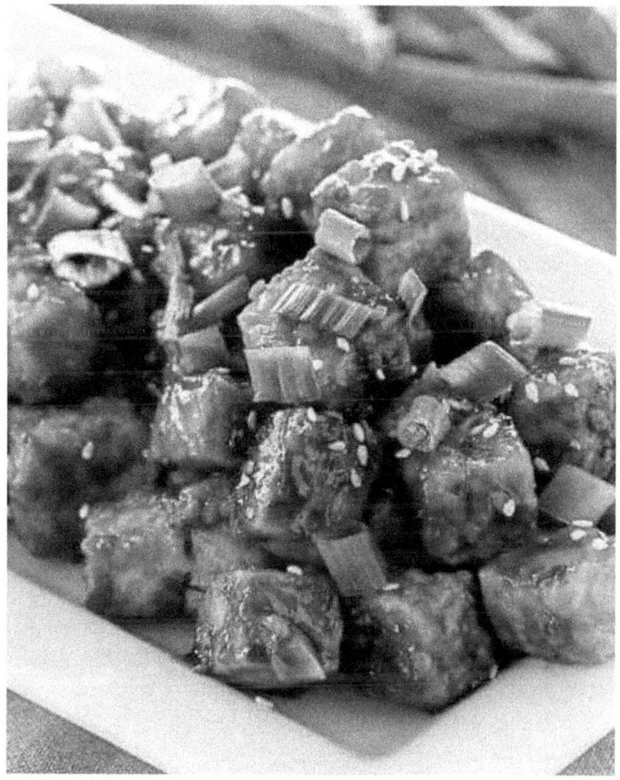

# Air Fryer Crab Cakes

**Prep Time: 10 minutes** **Cook Time: 14 minutes** **Servings: 11-12**

## INGREDIENTS

- 12 ounces canned lump crab meat, well drained
- 1/2 cup panko crumbs
- 1/4 cup diced celery
- 1 tablespoon chopped green onion
- 1 tablespoon mayonnaise
- 1 tablespoon extra virgin olive oil
- 1 large egg
- 1 1/2 teaspoons old bay seasoning
- 1/8 teaspoon kosher salt
- 1/8 teaspoon ground black pepper
- Cooking spray

## DIRECTIONS

1. Add all the ingredients to a large bowl and mix together until well combined. Cover and refrigerate for 30-60 minutes.
2. Portion out 3 tablespoons of the crab mixture and shape into a 1/2-inch thick patty. Repeat with remaining mixture. You should get 11-12 patties.
3. Spray the bottom of the air fryer basket with non-stick cooking spray. Place the patties in the air fryer basket and spray the tops with cooking spray or oil.
4. Air fry at 400F for 12-14 minutes, or until golden brown and crispy on the outside. (Depending on the size of your air fryer, you may need to air fry the crab cakes in two batches).
5. Serve hot and crispy with a squeeze of lemon and tartar sauce or herb dip.

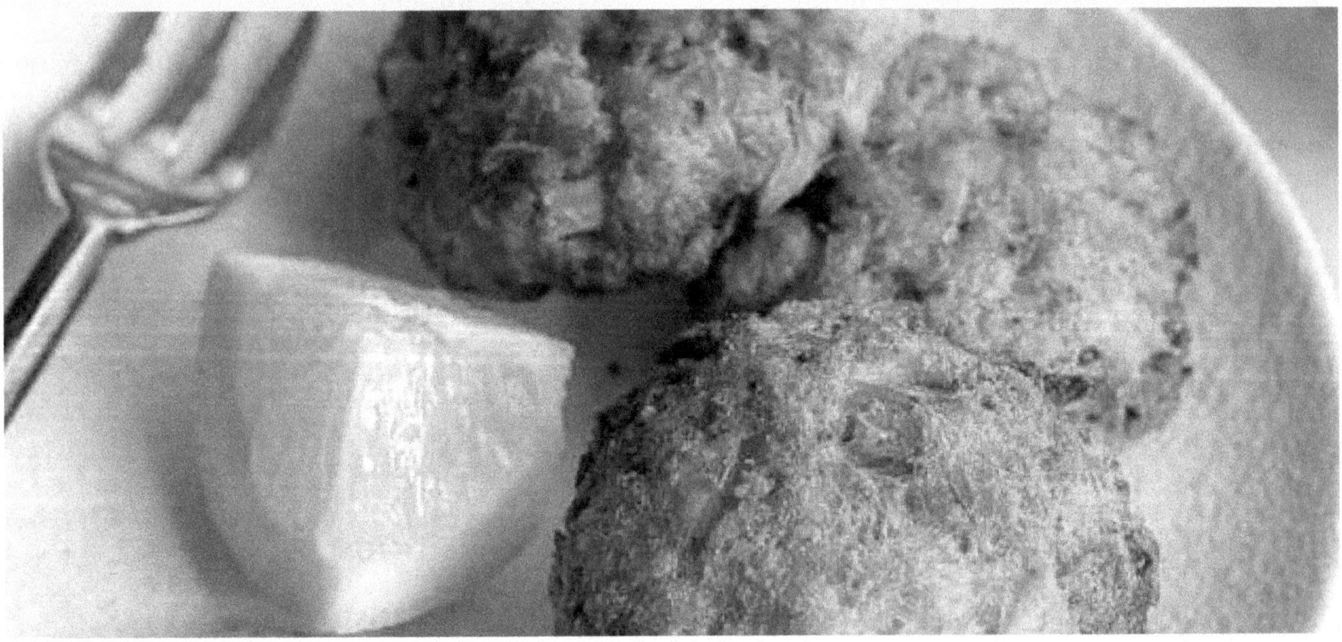

# Air Fryer Cajun Scallops

**Prep Time: 5 minutes** **Cook Time: 6 minutes** **Servings: 2**

**INGREDIENTS**

- 4-6 Sea scallops
- Cooking spray
- Kosher salt to taste
- Cajun seasoning

**DIRECTIONS**

1. Preheat your air fryer to 400 F.
2. Take your fresh sea scallops out of the fridge and quickly rinse them in cold water. Remove the side muscle with your fingers and pat dry with paper towels.
3. Once your air fryer is preheated, line the basket with aluminium foil and lightly spray with cooking spray.
4. Lightly spray the scallops with cooking oil and season with kosher salt and coat with cajun seasoning all over.
5. Place all the scallops in the air fryer and cook for 3 minutes. Flip and cook for 3 more minutes until they are opaque and register at least 130 F internally.
6. Serve with pasta, salad or alongside roasted vegetables.

◇◇◇◇◇◇◇◇◇◇◇◇◇◇◇◇◇◇◇◇◇◇◇◇◇◇◇◇◇◇◇◇◇◇◇◇◇◇◇◇

# Air Fryer Caramelized Bananas

**Prep time: 1 minutes** **Cook Time: 6 minutes** **Servings: 1**

**INGREDIENTS**

- 2 bananas
- 1/4 of a lemon, juiced
- 1 tbsp coconut sugar
- optonal toppings: cinnamon, nuts, coconut cream, yogurt, granola... etc.

**DIRECTIONS**

1. Wash your bananas with the peel on, then slice them straight down the middle, length wise
2. Squeeze lemon juice over top of each banana
3. If using cinnamon mix with in with the coconut sugar, then sprinkle over top of the bananas until coated
4. Place into parchment lined air fryer for 6-8 minutes at 400F
5. Once taken out of the airfryer, eat as is or top with your favourite toppings and enjoy!

# Air Fryer Sweet Chili Chicken Wings

**Prep Time: 10 minutes  Cook Time: 20 minutes  Servings: 2**

## INGREDIENTS

**Air Fryer Chicken Wings**

- 12 Chicken Wings
- 1/2 Tbsp Baking Powder NOT BAKING SODA
- 1 Tsp Ground Black Pepper
- 1/2 Tsp Sea Salt
- 1 Tsp Garlic Powder
- 1/4 Tsp Onion Powder
- 1/4 Tsp Paprika

**Thai Sweet Chili Sauce**

- 1 Tbsp Soy Sauce
- 1 1/2 Tbsp Hoisin Sauce
- 3 1/2 Tbsp Sweet Chili Sauce
- 1/2 Tbsp Rice Wine Vinegar
- 1/2 Tbsp Sesame Oil
- 1 Tbsp Brown Sugar Optional
- 2 Cloves Garlic Minced
- 1/2 Tsp Ground Ginger
- 1/4 Tsp Sea Salt
- 1/2 Tbsp Lime Juice
- 1/4 Cup Water

**Sriracha Ranch Dip**

- 1/3 Cup Homemade Buttermilk Ranch Dressing Or your favorite store bought brand
- 1 Tbsp Sriracha
- 1/4 Tsp Cayenne Pepper
- Optional Garnish
- Sesame Seeds
- Lime Juice
- Sliced Green Onion
- Cilantro

## DIRECTIONS

**Crispy Chicken Wings**

1. Dab chicken wings with a paper towel to ensure they are dry. Add the chicken wings to a zip-lock bag with baking powder and spices. Close the bag (making sure all the air is out) and toss everything together until the wings are coated.
2. Spray the metal rack (or basket) insert with cooking spray and arrange the chicken wings in a single layer. Close the Ninja Foodi lid and hit AIR CRISP, then set the TEMP to 400 degrees F, then set the TIME to 20 minutes and hit START. While the chicken wings are cooking make the sweet chili sauce.
3. *See Recipe Notes for oven instructions!
4. At 10 minutes open the lid and toss/flip the chicken wings with tongs to avoid them from sticking. Close the lid and allow them to cook for the remaining 10 minutes.
5. Once the time has expired check the internal temperature to ensure they are cooked though. Allow them to rest for 5 minutes before tossing in the sweet chili sauce.

**Sweet Chili Sauce**

6. Combine all ingredients into a small saucepan and heat over medium heat on the stove. Bring the sauce to a boil then reduce heat to a simmer stirring until the sauce has reduced and has slightly thickened. Keep sauce warm until chicken wings are finished.
7. Toss or dip the cooked chicken wings in the sauce. I like to make sure they are thoroughly coated.
8. Place the sauced chicken wings in a single layer on a greased cookie sheet with wire rack insert. Broil the chicken wings on the top rack on HIGH for 2-4 minutes. Stick close to the oven and check the wings often, they can burn quickly! Once the sauce is sticky and the wings have some color remove them from the oven. Serve warm with optional garnishes and Sriracha Ranch.

**Sriracha Ranch Dip**

9. Combine all ingredients in a small bowl and stir to combine. Serve with warm Sweet Chili Chicken Wings.

# Air Fryer Stuffed Peppers

**Prep Time: 5 minutes  Cook Time: 25 minutes  Servings: 6**

## INGREDIENTS

- 2 tablespoons olive oil
- 1 small yellow onion diced
- 2 cloves garlic minced
- 6 bell peppers (any color)
- 1 lb ground beef
- 2 1/2 teaspoons Italian seasoning
- 1 teaspoon salt
- 1 (15 ounce) can diced tomatoes (not drained)
- 1 tablespoon coconut aminos or Worcestershire sauce
- 1 cup uncooked white or brown rice
- 1 cup water
- 1 cup shredded cheddar cheese or vegan cheese (optional)

## DIRECTIONS

1. Preheat the air fryer to 400°F for 3-5 minutes. If your air fryer is smaller pre-heat for 3 minutes and if it's larger pre-heat for 5 minutes.
2. While it's heating, cut the tops off the peppers and scoop out any seeds. Dice the tops of the peppers and set aside to use in the mixture. When the air fryer is preheated, place the peppers in the basket of the air fryer and cook for 6 minutes.
3. While the peppers are cooking, make the filling. Heat the olive oil in a large and deep skillet over medium high heat. Once the olive oil is hot, add the onion and leftover diced peppers and cook for 2-3 minutes until soft and translucent. Add the garlic and cook for another 1-2 minutes until fragrant. Add the ground beef and brown until no pink remains (it should reach an internal temperature of 160°F).
4. Add the Italian seasoning, salt, diced tomatoes and coconut aminos (or worcestershire sauce) and stir to combine. Add the uncooked rice and water and stir. Turn the heat to medium low, cover the pot with the lid and simmer for 10-15 minutes, until the rice is tender.
5. When the beef and rice mixture is done scoop it evenly into each of the partially cooked peppers and place the peppers back in the air fryer. Air fry at 400°F for 4 minutes then open the drawer, top with shredded cheese and cook for another 4 minutes until melted and bubbly. If you aren't using cheese just air fry for 8 minutes.

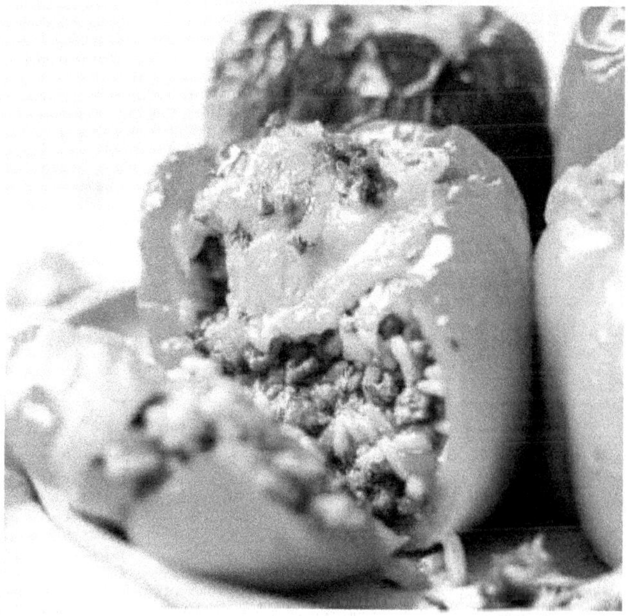

# Air Fryer Breakfast Burritos

**Prep Time: 15 minutes    Cook Time: 5 minutes    Servings: 6**

### INGREDIENTS

- 6 medium flour tortillas
- 6 scrambled eggs
- 1/2 lb ground sausage – browned
- 1/2 bell pepper – minced
- 1/3 cup bacon bits
- 1/2 cup shredded cheese
- oil for spraying

### DIRECTIONS

1. Combine scrambled eggs, cooked sausage, bell pepper, bacon bits & cheese in a large bowl. Stir to combine.
2. Spoon about 1/2 cup of the mixture into the center of a flour tortilla.
3. Fold in the sides & then roll.
4. Repeat with remaining ingredients.
5. Place filled burritos into the air fryer basket & spray liberally with oil.
6. Cook at 330 degrees for 5 minutes.

◇◇◇◇◇◇◇◇◇◇◇◇◇◇◇◇◇◇◇◇◇◇◇◇◇◇◇◇◇◇◇◇◇◇◇◇◇◇◇◇

# Air Fryer Turkey Breast

**Prep Time: 5 minutes    Cook Time: 45 minutes    Servings: 10**

### INGREDIENTS

- 3-4 pound bone-in turkey breast
- 2 tablespoons olive oil
- 1/2 tablespoon poultry seasoning
- 1 teaspoon ground sage
- 1 teaspoon ground thyme
- salt and pepper to taste

### DIRECTIONS

1. Rub the olive oil over both sides of the turkey breast. Sprinkle the seasonings onto both sides and rub them into the turkey.
2. Place the turkey skin-side down in the air fryer. Air fry for 25 minutes on 350 degrees.
3. Open the air fryer and flip the turkey. Cook for an additional 20-30 minutes. Test the thickest part of the turkey breast using a meat thermometer. Ensure the turkey has reached an internal temperature of 165 degrees. Mine was finished right at 45 minutes of total cook time.
4. Allow the turkey to rest for at least 10 minutes before slicing.

# Air Fryer Fish Tacos

**Prep Time: 20 minutes Cook Time: 12 minutes Servings: 4**

## INGREDIENTS

- 24 oz firm white fish fillets
- 1 tbsp grill seasoning
- 1 large avocado peeled and chopped
- 2 medium oranges peeled and chopped
- 1/4 cup red onion finely chopped
- 2 tbsp fresh cilantro finely chopped
- 1 tsp salt divided
- 1/4 cup mayonnaise
- 1/4 cup chipotle sauce
- 1 tbsp fresh lime juice
- corn tortillas

## DIRECTIONS

1. Stir together the avocado, orange, onion, cilantro and half teaspoon of salt. Set aside.
2. Stir together the mayonnaise, chipotle sauce, lime juice and remaining half teaspoon of salt. Set aside.
3. Evenly sprinkle the fish with the grill seasoning.
4. Brush the air fryer basket lightly with vegetable oil to prevent sticking.
5. Arrange the fish in a single layer in the basket. Cook at 400 degrees F for 8 - 12 minutes, or until the internal temperature of the fish reaches 145 degrees F. It is not necessary to flip the fish during cooking.
6. Serve the fish with warmed, corn tortillas, the avocado citrus salsa and chipotle mayonnaise to make tacos.

◇◇◇◇◇◇◇◇◇◇◇◇◇◇◇◇◇◇◇◇◇◇◇◇◇◇◇◇◇◇◇◇◇◇◇◇◇◇◇◇

# Air Fryer Sweet Potato Fries

**Prep Time: 5 minutes Cook Time: 12 minutes Servings: 2**

## INGREDIENTS

- 2 medium sweet potatoes peeled
- 2 teaspoons olive oil
- ½ teaspoon salt
- ¼ teaspoon garlic powder
- ¼ teaspoon paprika
- ⅛ teaspoon black pepper

## DIRECTIONS

1. Preheat the air fryer to 380°F. Peel the sweet potatoes, then slice each potato into even 1/4 inch thick sticks.
2. Place the sweet potatoes in a large mixing bowl, and toss with olive oil, salt, garlic powder, paprika and black pepper.
3. Cook in 2 or 3 batches, depending on the size of your basket without overcrowding the pan until they're crispy. I recommend 12 minutes, turning half way. This may vary based on your air fryer.
4. Serve immediately with your favorite dipping sauce.

# Air Fryer Potstickers

**Prep Time: 5 minutes  Cook Time: 10 minutes  Servings: 2**

## INGREDIENTS

**DUMPLINGS**

- 8 ounces frozen vegetable, pork, or chicken dumplings

**DIPPING SAUCE**

- 1/4 cup soy sauce
- 1/4 cup water
- 1/8 cup maple syrup (or molasses)
- 1/2 teaspoon garlic powder
- 1/2 teaspoon rice vinegar
- small pinch of red pepper flakes

## DIRECTIONS

1. Preheat your air fryer to 370 degrees for about 4 minutes.
2. Place the frozen dumplings inside the air fryer in one layer and spray with oil.
3. Cook for 5 minutes, shake the basket, then spray with a little more oil.
4. Cook dumplings for another 4-6 minutes.
5. Meanwhile, prepare the dipping sauce by mixing ingredients together.
6. Remove the air fryer dumplings from the basket and let sit for another 2 minutes before enjoying.

◇◇◇◇◇◇◇◇◇◇◇◇◇◇◇◇◇◇◇◇◇◇◇◇◇◇◇◇◇◇◇◇◇◇◇◇◇◇◇◇

# Air Fryer Chimichangas

**Prep Time: 17 minutes  Cook Time: 17 minutes  Servings: 8**

## INGREDIENTS

**For the Chicken:**

- 4 cups of deli-style cooked shredded rotisserie chicken or shredded chicken breast
- 1 large onion, finely chopped
- 1 4oz. can chopped green chilies
- 4 tbsp all-purpose flour
- 1 16 oz can of red enchilada sauce.
- ¼ tsp garlic powder
- 1 tsp ground cuminutes
- 8 (6 in) flour tortillas
- Toppings for Chimichangas (optional)
- Reduced Fat Cheddar Cheese
- Plain Greek Yogurt
- Cilantro or Scallions

## DIRECTIONS

1. Preheat air fryer to 400°F. Coat a large skillet with cooking spray.
2. Add onions and green chilies to pan and saute for 2 minutes. When the onions are soft add flour, salt, cumin, garlic powder, enchilada sauce, and continue stirring. When the sauce has thickened add in precooked shredded chicken. If the sauce looks too thick add in some chicken stock to thin it out. (2 tablespoons to start)
3. Take off heat and begin preparing the chimichangas for cooking them in the air fryer.
4. Assemble chimichangas by spooning about 1/2 cup of chicken mixture onto each tortilla; fold in sides and roll up.
5. Spray the outside of each filled tortilla with cooking spray; place 4 in the basket of air fryer, seam side down. Set to 400°F; cook 4 minutes. Turn; cook 2 to 3 minutes or until lightly browned and heated through. Repeat with remaining 4 filled tortillas.

# Crispy Air Fryer Bacon

**Prep Time: 2 minutes  Cook Time: 8 minutes  Servings: 12**

## INGREDIENTS

- 1 package of thick cut bacon

## DIRECTIONS

1. Line the outer basket with aluminum foil and pre-heat the air fryer to 390° F. You can also add 1-2 slices of bread to the bottom basket to soak up the grease.
2. Cut the bacon slices in half (or don't, this is optional) and arrange them in the basket in a flat layer. Cook the bacon 5 minutes, then flip and cook for another 3-4 minutes depending on how you like your bacon. If you like it extra crispy, cook it for 4-5 minutes after flipping (total time 8-10 minutes). When finished, remove the bacon strips from the air fryer and transfer to a paper towel lined plate.

◇◇◇◇◇◇◇◇◇◇◇◇◇◇◇◇◇◇◇◇◇◇◇◇◇◇◇◇◇◇◇◇◇◇◇◇◇◇◇◇◇

# Air Fryer Chicken Parmesan

**Prep Time: 10 minutes  Cook Time: 15 minutes  Servings: 3**

## INGREDIENTS

- 3 chicken breasts medium size, thawed
- 2 eggs whisked
- 1/4 c bread crumbs
- 1/4 c parmesan cheese
- 1/2 tsp onion powder
- 1/2 tsp Italian seasoning
- 1/2 tsp garlic powder
- 1/2 c marinara sauce
- 1/2 c mozzarella cheese shredded, or more

## DIRECTIONS

1. In a small bowl whisk eggs, in another bowl combine bread crumbs, parmesan, and onion and garlic powder.
2. Dredge chicken breast in egg, then cover in bread crumb mixture generously shaking off excess. (make sure breasts are about med. size and are all similar sizes so they cook evenly)
3. Spray inside of air fryer basket with non stick spray and put coated breasts inside.
4. Close and set air fryer to 360 degrees for 15-18 minutes. Cook time will depend on thickness of chicken.
5. Open basket and spoon marinara sauce over cooked breasts, then sprinkle with cheese. Air fry for additional 2 minutes until cheese is melted.
6. Sprinkle top with Italian seasonings and serve!

# AIR-FRYER RECIPES YOU NEED TO TRY

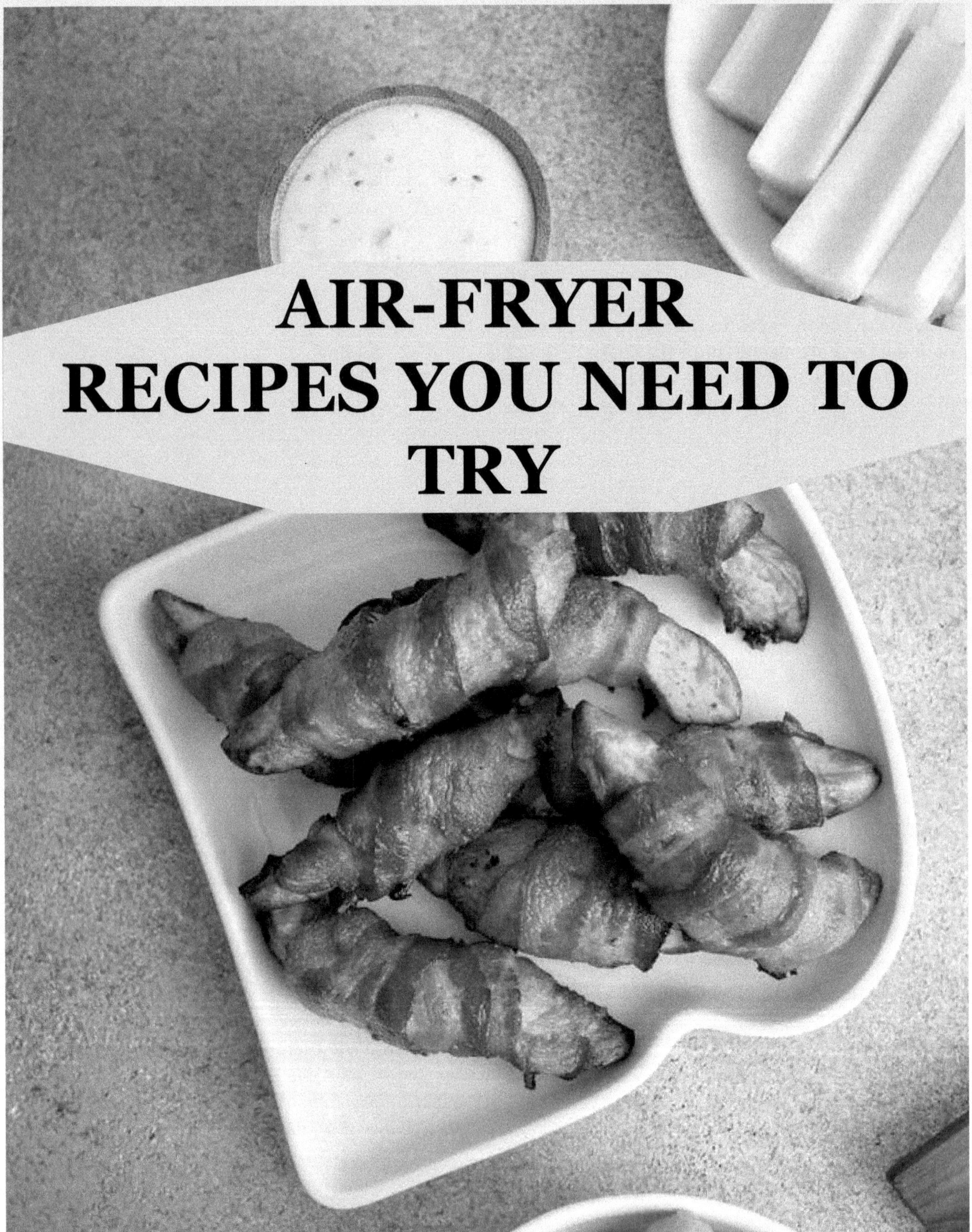

# Air-Fryer Coconut Shrimp and Apricot Sauce

**TOTAL TIME: Prep: 25 min. Cook: 10 min./batch    Servings: 6**

**INGREDIENTS**

- 1-1/2 pounds uncooked shrimp (26-30 per pound)
- 1-1/2 cups sweetened shredded coconut
- 1/2 cup panko bread crumbs
- 4 large egg whites
- 3 dashes Louisiana-style hot sauce
- 1/4 teaspoon salt
- 1/4 teaspoon pepper
- 1/2 cup all-purpose flour

**SAUCE:**

- 1 cup apricot preserves
- 1 teaspoon cider vinegar
- 1/4 teaspoon crushed red pepper flakes

**DIRECTIONS**

1. Preheat air fryer to 375°. Peel and devein shrimp, leaving tails on.
2. In a shallow bowl, toss coconut with bread crumbs. In another shallow bowl, whisk egg whites, hot sauce, salt and pepper. Place flour in a third shallow bowl.
3. Dip shrimp in flour to coat lightly; shake off excess. Dip in egg white mixture, then in coconut mixture, patting to help coating adhere.
4. In batches, place shrimp in a single layer on greased tray in air-fryer basket. Cook 4 minutes. Turn shrimp; cook until coconut is lightly browned and shrimp turn pink, about 4 minutes longer.
5. Meanwhile, combine sauce ingredients in a small saucepan; cook and stir over medium-low heat until preserves are melted. Serve shrimp immediately with sauce.

◇◇◇◇◇◇◇◇◇◇◇◇◇◇◇◇◇◇◇◇◇◇◇◇◇◇◇◇◇◇◇◇◇◇◇◇◇◇◇◇

# Air-Fryer Garlic-Rosemary Brussels Sprouts

**TOTAL TIME: 30 min.    Servings: 4**

**INGREDIENTS**

- 3 tablespoons olive oil
- 2 garlic cloves, minced
- 1/2 teaspoon salt
- 1/4 teaspoon pepper
- 1 pound Brussels sprouts, trimmed and halved
- 1/2 cup panko bread crumbs
- 1-1/2 teaspoons minced fresh rosemary

**DIRECTIONS**

1. Preheat air fryer to 350°. Place first 4 ingredients in a small microwave-safe bowl; microwave on high 30 seconds.
2. Toss Brussels sprouts with 2 tablespoons oil mixture. Place Brussels sprouts on tray in air-fryer basket; cook 4-5 minutes. Stir sprouts. Cook until sprouts are lightly browned and near desired tenderness, about 8 minutes longer, stirring halfway through cooking time.
3. Toss bread crumbs with rosemary and remaining oil mixture; sprinkle over sprouts. Continue cooking until crumbs are browned and sprouts are tender, 3-5 minutes. Serve immediately.

# Air-Fryer Stuffed Sweet Potatoes

**TOTAL TIME: Prep: 20 min. Cook: 45 min. Servings: 4**

**INGREDIENTS**

- 2 medium sweet potatoes
- 1 teaspoon olive oil
- 1 cup cooked chopped spinach, drained
- 1 cup shredded cheddar cheese, divided
- 2 cooked bacon strips, crumbled
- 1 green onion, chopped
- 1/4 cup fresh cranberries, coarsely chopped
- 1/3 cup chopped pecans, toasted
- 2 tablespoons butter
- 1/4 teaspoon kosher salt
- 1/4 teaspoon pepper

**DIRECTIONS**

1. Preheat air fryer to 400°. Brush potatoes with oil. Place on tray in air-fryer basket. Cook until potatoes are tender, 30-40 minutes; cool slightly.
2. Cut potatoes in half lengthwise. Scoop out pulp, leaving a 1/4-inch thick shell. In a large bowl, mash the potato pulp; stir in spinach, 3/4 cup cheese, bacon, onion, cranberries, pecans, butter, salt and pepper. Spoon into potato shells, mounding slightly.
3. Reduce heat to 360°. Place potato halves, cut side up, on tray in air-fryer basket. Cook 10 minutes. Sprinkle with remaining 1/4 cup cheese; cook until cheese is melted, 1-2 minutes.

◇◇◇◇◇◇◇◇◇◇◇◇◇◇◇◇◇◇◇◇◇◇◇◇◇◇◇◇◇◇◇◇◇◇◇◇◇◇◇◇◇◇◇◇◇◇◇◇◇◇◇◇

# Popcorn Shrimp Tacos with Cabbage Slaw

**TOTAL TIME: Prep/Total Time: 30 min. Servings: 4**

**INGREDIENTS**

- 2 cups coleslaw mix
- 1/4 cup minced fresh cilantro
- 2 tablespoons lime juice
- 2 tablespoons honey
- 1/4 teaspoon salt
- 1 jalapeno pepper, seeded and minced, optional
- 2 large eggs
- 2 tablespoons 2% milk
- 1/2 cup all-purpose flour
- 1-1/2 cups panko bread crumbs
- 1 tablespoon ground cumin
- 1 tablespoon garlic powder
- 1 pound uncooked shrimp (41-50 per pound), peeled and deveined
- Cooking spray
- 8 corn tortillas (6 inches), warmed
- 1 medium ripe avocado, peeled and sliced

**DIRECTIONS**

1. In a small bowl, combine coleslaw mix, cilantro, lime juice, honey, salt and, if desired, jalapeno; toss to coat. Set aside.
2. Preheat air fryer to 375°. In a shallow bowl, whisk eggs and milk. Place flour in a separate shallow bowl. In a third shallow bowl, mix panko, cumin and garlic powder. Dip shrimp in flour to coat both sides; shake off excess. Dip in egg mixture, then in panko mixture, patting to help coating adhere.
3. In batches, arrange shrimp in a single layer on greased tray in air-fryer basket; spritz with cooking spray. Cook until golden brown, 2-3 minutes. Turn; spritz with cooking spray. Cook until golden brown and shrimp turn pink, 2-3 minutes longer.
4. Serve shrimp in tortillas with coleslaw mix and avocado.

# Bacon-Wrapped Avocado Wedges

**TOTAL TIME: Prep/Total Time: 30 min. Servings: 1**

## INGREDIENTS

- 2 medium ripe avocados
- 12 bacon strips

**SAUCE:**

- 1/2 cup mayonnaise
- 2 to 3 tablespoons Sriracha chili sauce
- 1 to 2 tablespoons lime juice
- 1 teaspoon grated lime zest

## DIRECTIONS

1. Preheat air fryer to 400°. Cut each avocado in half; remove pit and peel. Cut each half into thirds. Wrap 1 bacon slice around each avocado wedge. Working in batches if needed, place wedges in a single layer on tray in air-fryer basket and cook until bacon is cooked through, 10-15 minutes.
2. Meanwhile, in a small bowl, stir together mayonnaise, Sriracha sauce, lime juice and zest. Serve wedges with sauce.

# Air-Fryer Steak Fajitas

**TOTAL TIME: Prep/Total Time: 30 min. Servings: 6**

## INGREDIENTS

- 2 large tomatoes, seeded and chopped
- 1/2 cup diced red onion
- 1/4 cup lime juice
- 1 jalapeno pepper, seeded and minced
- 3 tablespoons minced fresh cilantro
- 2 teaspoons ground cumin, divided
- 3/4 teaspoon salt, divided
- 1 beef flank steak (about 1-1/2 pounds)
- 1 large onion, halved and sliced
- 6 whole wheat tortillas (8 inches), warmed
- Optional: Sliced avocado and lime wedges

## DIRECTIONS

1. For salsa, place first 5 ingredients in a small bowl; stir in 1 teaspoon cumin and 1/4 teaspoon salt. Let stand until serving.
2. Preheat air fryer to 400°. Sprinkle steak with the remaining cumin and salt. Place on greased tray in air-fryer basket. Cook until meat reaches desired doneness (for medium-rare, a thermometer should read 135°; medium, 140°; medium-well, 145°), 6-8 minutes per side. Remove from basket and let stand 5 minutes.
3. Meanwhile, place onion on tray in air-fryer basket. Cook until crisp-tender, 2-3 minutes, stirring once. Slice steak thinly across the grain; serve in tortillas with onion and salsa. If desired, serve with avocado and lime wedges.

# Air-Fryer Coconut Shrimp

**TOTAL TIME: Prep/Total Time: 30 min.     Servings: 2**

## INGREDIENTS

- 1/2 pound uncooked large shrimp
- 1/2 cup sweetened shredded coconut
- 3 tablespoons panko bread crumbs
- 2 large egg whites
- 1/8 teaspoon salt
- Dash pepper
- Dash Louisiana-style hot sauce
- 3 tablespoons all-purpose flour
- SAUCE:
- 1/3 cup apricot preserves
- 1/2 teaspoon cider vinegar
- Dash crushed red pepper flakes

## DIRECTIONS

1. Preheat air fryer to 375°. Peel and devein shrimp, leaving tails on.
2. In a shallow bowl, toss coconut with bread crumbs. In another shallow bowl, whisk egg whites, salt, pepper and hot sauce. Place flour in a third shallow bowl.
3. Dip shrimp in flour to coat lightly; shake off excess. Dip in egg white mixture, then in coconut mixture, patting to help coating adhere.
4. Place shrimp in a single layer on greased tray in air-fryer basket. Cook 4 minutes; turn shrimp and continue cooking until coconut is lightly browned and shrimp turn pink, about 4 minutes longer.
5. Meanwhile, combine sauce ingredients in a small saucepan; cook and stir over medium-low heat until preserves are melted. Serve shrimp immediately with sauce.

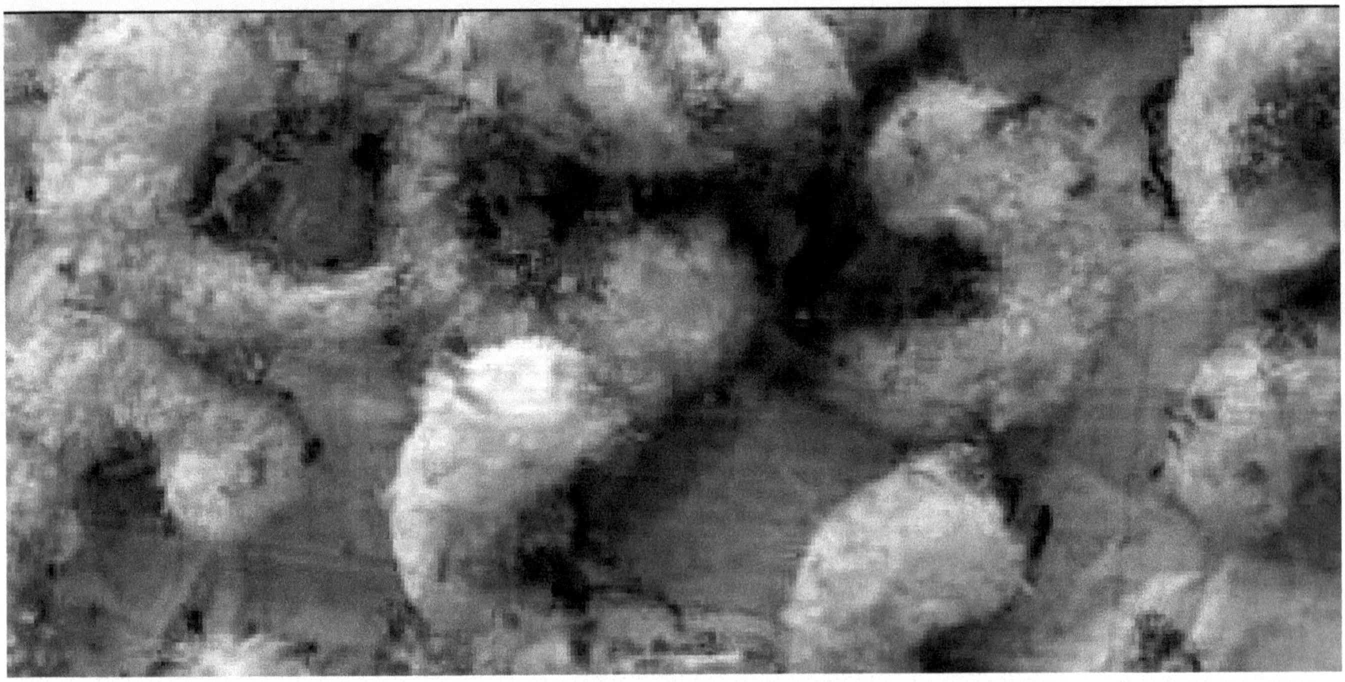

# Sweet and Spicy Air-Fryer Meatballs

**TOTAL TIME: Prep: 30 min. Cook: 15 min./batch    Servings: 3**

**INGREDIENTS**

- 2/3 cup quick-cooking oats
- 1/2 cup crushed Ritz crackers
- 2 large eggs, lightly beaten
- 1 can (5 ounces) evaporated milk
- 1 tablespoon dried minced onion
- 1 teaspoon salt
- 1 teaspoon garlic powder
- 1 teaspoon ground cumin
- 1 teaspoon honey
- 1/2 teaspoon pepper
- 2 pounds lean ground beef (90% lean)

**SAUCE:**

- 1/3 cup packed brown sugar
- 1/3 cup honey
- 1/3 cup orange marmalade
- 2 tablespoons cornstarch
- 2 tablespoons soy sauce
- 1 to 2 tablespoons Louisiana-style hot sauce
- 1 tablespoon Worcestershire sauce

**DIRECTIONS**

1. Preheat air fryer to 380°. In a large bowl, combine the first 10 ingredients. Add beef; mix lightly but thoroughly. Shape into 1-1/2-in. balls.
2. In batches, arrange meatballs in a single layer on greased tray in air-fryer basket. Cook until they are lightly browned and cooked through, 12-15 minutes. Meanwhile, in a small saucepan, combine sauce ingredients. Cook and stir over medium heat until thickened. Serve with meatballs.

# Air-Fryer Chocolate Chip Oatmeal Cookies

**TOTAL TIME: Prep: 20 min. Cook: 10 min./batch    Servings: 6**

**INGREDIENTS**

- 1 cup butter, softened
- 3/4 cup sugar
- 3/4 cup packed brown sugar
- 2 large eggs, room temperature
- 1 teaspoon vanilla extract
- 3 cups quick-cooking oats
- 1-1/2 cups all-purpose flour
- 1 package (3.4 ounces) instant vanilla pudding mix
- 1 teaspoon baking soda
- 1 teaspoon salt
- 2 cups semisweet chocolate chips
- 1 cup chopped nuts

**DIRECTIONS**

1. Preheat air fryer to 325°. In a large bowl, cream butter and sugars until light and fluffy, 5-7 minutes. Beat in eggs and vanilla. In another bowl, whisk oats, flour, dry pudding mix, baking soda and salt; gradually beat into creamed mixture. Stir in chocolate chips and nuts.
2. Drop dough by tablespoonfuls onto baking sheets; flatten slightly. In batches, place 1 in. apart on greased tray in air-fryer basket. Cook until lightly browned, 8-10 minutes. Remove to wire racks to cool.

# Air-Fryer Calamari

**TOTAL TIME: Prep Time: 20 min. Cook Time: 10 min./batch Servings: 5**

## INGREDIENTS

- 1/2 cup all-purpose flour
- 1/2 teaspoon salt
- 1 large egg, lightly beaten
- 1/2 cup 2% milk
- 1 cup panko bread crumbs
- 1/2 teaspoon seasoned salt
- 1/4 teaspoon pepper
- 8 ounces cleaned fresh or frozen calamari (squid), thawed and cut into 1/2-inch rings
- Cooking spray

## DIRECTIONS

1. Preheat air fryer to 400°. In a shallow bowl, combine flour and salt. In another shallow bowl, whisk egg and milk. In a third shallow bowl, combine bread crumbs, seasoned salt and pepper. Coat calamari with flour mixture, then dip in egg mixture and coat with bread crumb mixture.
2. In batches, place calamari in a single layer on greased tray in air-fryer basket; spritz with cooking spray. Cook 4 minutes. Turn; spritz with cooking spray. Cook until golden brown, 3-5 minutes longer.

◇◇◇◇◇◇◇◇◇◇◇◇◇◇◇◇◇◇◇◇◇◇◇◇◇◇◇◇◇◇◇◇◇◇◇◇◇◇◇◇

# Air-Fryer Ravioli

**TOTAL TIME: Prep: 20 min. Cook: 10 min./batch Servings: 1-1/2**

## INGREDIENTS

- 1 cup seasoned bread crumbs
- 1/4 cup shredded Parmesan cheese
- 2 teaspoons dried basil
- 1/2 cup all-purpose flour
- 2 large eggs, lightly beaten
- 1 package (9 ounces) frozen beef ravioli, thawed
- Cooking spray
- Fresh minced basil, optional
- 1 cup marinara sauce, warmed

## DIRECTIONS

1. Preheat air fryer to 350°. In a shallow bowl, mix bread crumbs, Parmesan cheese and basil. Place flour and eggs in separate shallow bowls. Dip ravioli in flour to coat both sides; shake off excess. Dip in eggs, then in crumb mixture, patting to help coating adhere.
2. In batches, arrange ravioli in a single layer on greased tray in air-fryer basket; spritz with cooking spray. Cook until golden brown, 3-4 minutes. Turn; spritz with cooking spray. Cook until golden brown, 3-4 minutes longer. If desired, immediately sprinkle with basil and additional Parmesan cheese. Serve warm with marinara sauce.

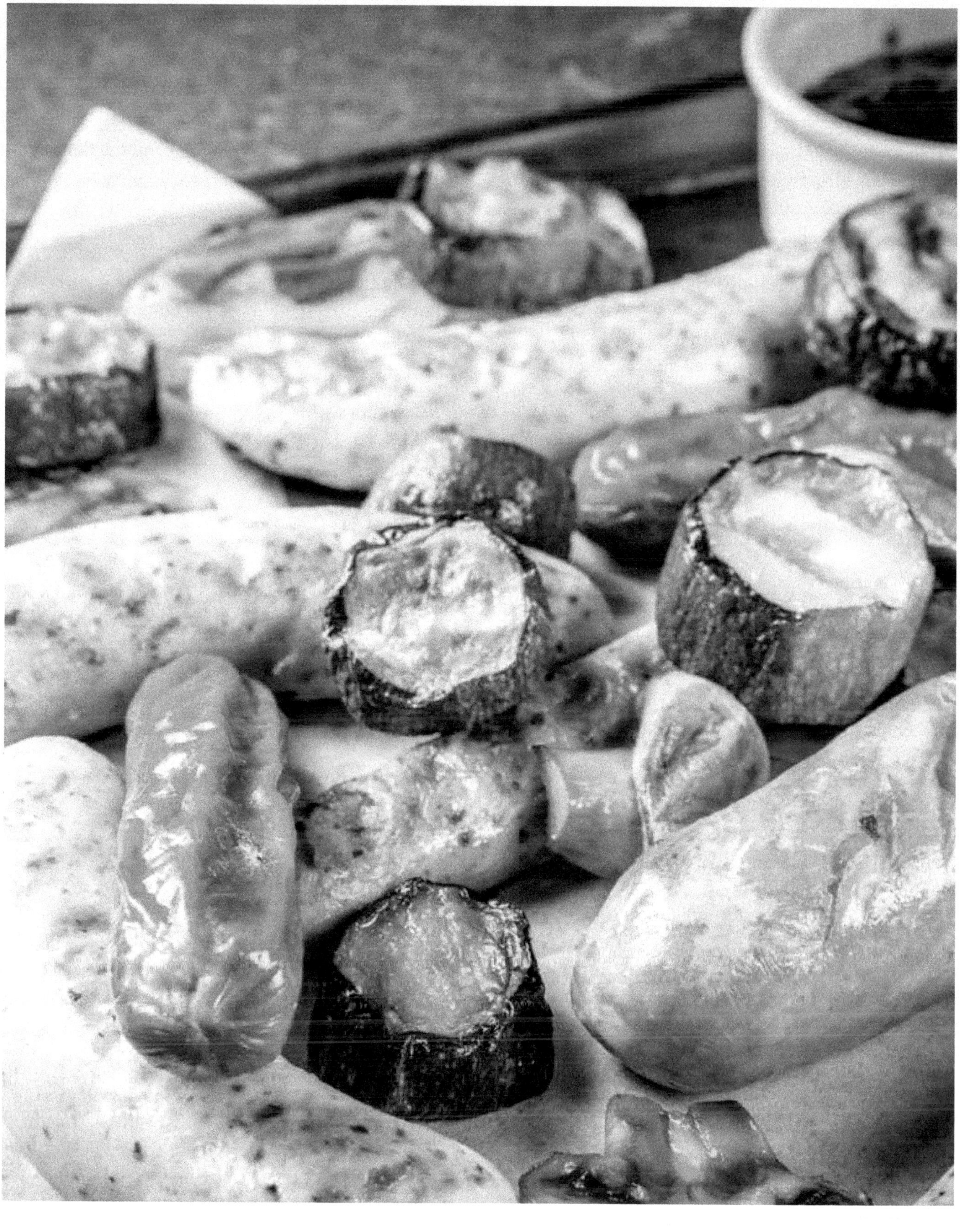

# Air-Fryer Pickles

**TOTAL TIME: Prep: 20 min. + standing Cook: 15 min./batch Servings: 32**

## INGREDIENTS

- 32 dill pickle slices
- 1/2 cup all-purpose flour
- 1/2 teaspoon salt
- 3 large eggs, lightly beaten
- 2 tablespoons dill pickle juice
- 1/2 teaspoon cayenne pepper
- 1/2 teaspoon garlic powder
- 2 cups panko bread crumbs
- 2 tablespoons snipped fresh dill
- Cooking spray
- Ranch salad dressing, optional

## DIRECTIONS

1. Preheat air fryer to 400°. Let pickles stand on paper towels until liquid is almost absorbed, about 15 minutes.
2. Meanwhile, in a shallow bowl, combine flour and salt. In another shallow bowl, whisk eggs, pickle juice, cayenne and garlic powder. Combine panko and dill in a third shallow bowl.
3. Dip pickles in flour mixture to coat both sides; shake off excess. Dip in egg mixture, then in crumb mixture, patting to help coating adhere. In batches, place pickles in a single layer on greased tray in air-fryer basket. Cook until golden brown and crispy, 7-10 minutes. Turn pickles; spritz with cooking spray. Cook until golden brown and crispy, 7-10 minutes longer. Serve immediately, with ranch dressing if desired.

◇◇◇◇◇◇◇◇◇◇◇◇◇◇◇◇◇◇◇◇◇◇◇◇◇◇◇◇◇◇◇◇◇◇◇◇◇◇◇◇◇◇◇◇

# Air-Fryer Fish and Fries

**TOTAL TIME: Prep: 15 min. Cook: 25 min. Servings: 4**

## INGREDIENTS

- 1 pound potatoes (about 2 medium)
- 2 tablespoons olive oil
- 1/4 teaspoon pepper
- 1/4 teaspoon salt

**FISH:**

- 1/3 cup all-purpose flour
- 1/4 teaspoon pepper
- 1 large egg, room temperature
- 2 tablespoons water
- 2/3 cup crushed cornflakes
- 1 tablespoon grated Parmesan cheese
- 1/8 teaspoon cayenne pepper
- 1 pound haddock or cod fillets
- 1/4 teaspoon salt
- Tartar sauce, optional

## DIRECTIONS

1. Preheat air fryer to 400°. Peel and cut potatoes lengthwise into 1/2-in.-thick slices; cut slices into 1/2-in.-thick sticks.
2. In a large bowl, toss potatoes with oil, pepper and salt. Working in batches, place potatoes in a single layer on tray in air-fryer basket; cook until just tender, 5-10 minutes Toss potatoes to redistribute; cook until lightly browned and crisp, 5-10 minutes longer.
3. Meanwhile, in a shallow bowl, mix flour and pepper. In another shallow bowl, whisk egg with water. In a third bowl, toss cornflakes with cheese and cayenne. Sprinkle fish with salt. Dip into flour mixture to coat both sides; shake off excess. Dip in egg mixture, then in cornflake mixture, patting to help coating adhere.
4. Remove fries from basket; keep warm. Place fish in a single layer on tray in air-fryer basket. Cook until fish is lightly browned and just beginning to flake easily with a fork, 8-10 minutes, turning halfway through cooking. Do not overcook. Return fries to basket to heat through. Serve immediately. If desired, serve with tartar sauce.

# Air-Fryer Caribbean Wontons

**TOTAL TIME: Prep: 30 min. Cook: 10 min./batch Servings: 2**

## INGREDIENTS

- 4 ounces cream cheese, softened
- 1/4 cup sweetened shredded coconut
- 1/4 cup mashed ripe banana
- 2 tablespoons chopped walnuts
- 2 tablespoons canned crushed pineapple
- 1 cup marshmallow creme
- 24 wonton wrappers
- Cooking spray

**SAUCE:**

- 1 pound fresh strawberries, hulled
- 1/4 cup sugar
- 1 teaspoon cornstarch
- Confectioners' sugar and ground cinnamon

## DIRECTIONS

1. Preheat air fryer to 350°. In a small bowl, beat cream cheese until smooth. Stir in coconut, banana, walnuts and pineapple. Fold in marshmallow creme.
2. Position a wonton wrapper with 1 point toward you. Keep remaining wrappers covered with a damp paper towel until ready to use. Place 2 teaspoons filling in the center of wrapper. Moisten edges with water; fold opposite corners together over filling and press to seal. Repeat with remaining wrappers and filling.
3. In batches, arrange wontons in a single layer on greased tray in air-fryer basket; spritz with cooking spray. Cook until golden brown and crisp, 10-12 minutes.
4. Meanwhile, place strawberries in a food processor; cover and process until pureed. In a small saucepan, combine sugar and cornstarch. Stir in pureed strawberries. Bring to a boil; cook and stir until thickened, 2 minutes. If desired, strain mixture, reserving sauce; discard seeds. Sprinkle wontons with confectioners' sugar and cinnamon. Serve with sauce.

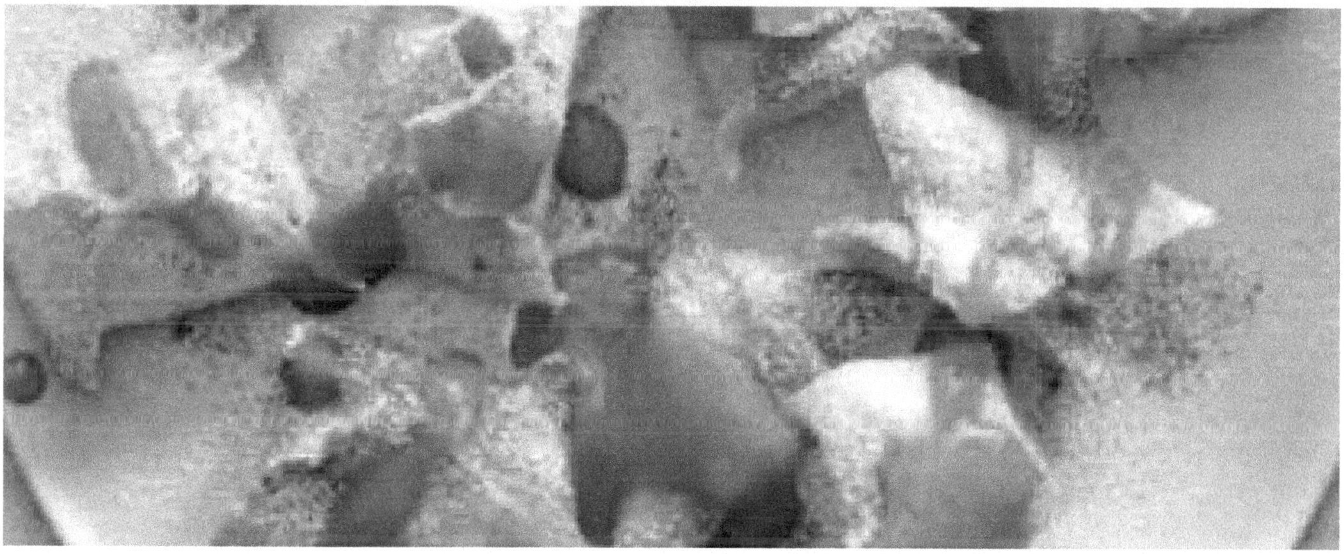

# Air-Fried Radishes

**TOTAL TIME: Prep/Total Time: 25 min.  Servings: 6**

## INGREDIENTS

- 2-1/4 pounds radishes, trimmed and quartered (about 6 cups)
- 3 tablespoons olive oil
- 1 tablespoon minced fresh oregano or 1 teaspoon dried oregano
- 1/4 teaspoon salt
- 1/8 teaspoon pepper

## DIRECTIONS

1. Preheat air fryer to 375°. Toss radishes with remaining ingredients. Place radishes on greased tray in air-fryer basket. Cook until crisp-tender, 12-15 minutes, stirring occasionally.

◇◇◇◇◇◇◇◇◇◇◇◇◇◇◇◇◇◇◇◇◇◇◇◇◇◇◇◇◇◇◇◇◇◇◇◇◇◇◇◇

# Air-Fryer Ham and Egg Pockets

**TOTAL TIME: Prep/Total Time: 25 min.  Servings: 2**

## INGREDIENTS

- 1 large egg
- 2 teaspoons 2% milk
- 2 teaspoons butter
- 1 ounce thinly sliced deli ham, chopped
- 2 tablespoons shredded cheddar cheese
- 1 tube (4 ounces) refrigerated crescent rolls

## DIRECTIONS

1. 1. Preheat air fryer to 300°. In a small bowl, combine egg and milk. In a small skillet, heat butter until hot. Add egg mixture; cook and stir over medium heat until eggs are completely set. Remove from the heat. Fold in ham and cheese.
2. 2. Separate crescent dough into 2 rectangles. Seal perforations; spoon half the filling down the center of each rectangle. Fold dough over filling; pinch to seal. Place in a single layer on greased tray in air-fryer basket. Cook until golden brown, 8-10 minutes.

# Air-Fryer Taco Twists

**TOTAL TIME: Prep: 15 min. Cook: 20 min. Servings: 4**

## INGREDIENTS

- 1/3 pound ground beef
- 1 large onion, chopped
- 2/3 cup shredded cheddar cheese
- 1/3 cup salsa
- 3 tablespoons canned chopped green chiles
- 1/4 teaspoon garlic powder
- 1/4 teaspoon hot pepper sauce
- 1/8 teaspoon salt
- 1/8 teaspoon ground cumin
- 1 tube (8 ounces) refrigerated crescent rolls
- Optional: Shredded lettuce, sliced ripe olives, chopped tomatoes and sliced seeded jalapeno pepper

## DIRECTIONS

1. Preheat air fryer to 300°. In a large skillet, cook beef and onion over medium heat until meat is no longer pink; crumble meat; drain. Stir in cheese, salsa, chiles, garlic powder, hot pepper sauce, salt and cumin.
2. Unroll crescent roll dough and separate into 4 rectangles; press perforations to seal. Place 1/2 cup meat mixture in the center of each rectangle. Bring 4 corners to the center and twist; pinch to seal. In batches, place in a single layer on greased tray in air-fryer basket. Cook until golden brown, 18-22 minutes. If desired, serve with toppings of your choice.

◇◇◇◇◇◇◇◇◇◇◇◇◇◇◇◇◇◇◇◇◇◇◇◇◇◇◇◇◇◇◇◇◇◇◇◇◇◇◇◇

# Air-Fryer Potato Chips

**TOTAL TIME: Prep: 20 min. + soaking Cook: 15 min./batch Servings: 6**

## INGREDIENTS

- 2 large potatoes
- Olive oil-flavored cooking spray
- 1/2 teaspoon sea salt
- Minced fresh parsley, optional

## DIRECTIONS

1. Preheat air fryer to 360°. Using a mandoline or vegetable peeler, cut potatoes into very thin slices. Transfer to a large bowl; add enough ice water to cover. Soak for 15 minutes; drain. Add more ice water and soak another 15 minutes.
2. Drain potatoes; place on towels and pat dry. Spritz potatoes with cooking spray; sprinkle with salt. In batches, place potato slices in a single layer on greased tray in air-fryer basket. Cook until crisp and golden brown, 15-17 minutes, stirring and turning every 5-7 minutes. If desired, sprinkle with parsley.

# Air-Fryer Spicy Ginger Beef Skewers

**TOTAL TIME: Prep: 20 min. + marinating Cook: 5 min. Servings: 6**

## INGREDIENTS

- 1 beef flank steak (1-1/2 pounds)
- 1 cup rice vinegar
- 1 cup soy sauce
- 1/4 cup packed brown sugar
- 2 tablespoons minced fresh gingerroot
- 6 garlic cloves, minced
- 3 teaspoons sesame oil
- 2 teaspoons Sriracha chili sauce or 1 teaspoon hot pepper sauce
- 1/2 teaspoon cornstarch
- Optional: Sesame seeds and thinly sliced green onions

## DIRECTIONS

1. Cut beef into 1/4-in.-thick strips. In a large bowl, whisk the next 7 ingredients until blended. Pour 1 cup marinade into a shallow dish. Add beef; turn to coat. Cover and refrigerate 2-8 hours. Cover and refrigerate remaining marinade.
2. Preheat air fryer to 400°. Drain beef, discarding marinade in dish. Thread beef onto 12 metal or soaked wooden skewers that fit into air fryer. Working in batches if necessary, arrange skewers in a single layer on greased tray in air-fryer basket. Cook until meat reaches desired doneness (for medium-rare, a thermometer should read 135°; medium, 140°; medium-well, 145°), 4-5 minutes, turning occasionally and basting frequently, using 1/2 cup of reserved marinade.
3. Meanwhile, to make glaze, bring remaining marinade (about 3/4 cup) to a boil; whisk in 1/2 teaspoon cornstarch. Cook, whisking constantly, until thickened, 1-2 minutes. Brush skewers with glaze just before serving. If desired, top with sesame seeds and sliced green onions.

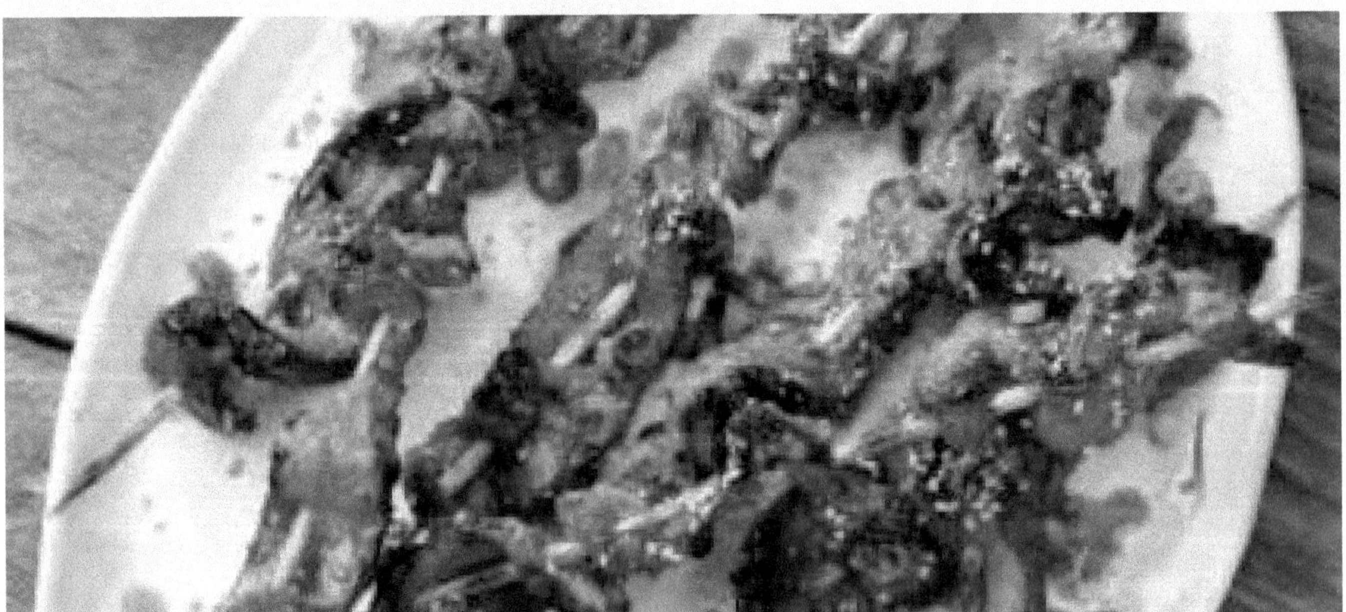

# Air-Fryer Carrot Coffee Cake

**TOTAL TIME: Prep: 15 min. Bake: 35 min. Servings: 6**

## INGREDIENTS

- 1 large egg, lightly beaten, room temperature
- 1/2 cup buttermilk
- 1/3 cup sugar plus 2 tablespoons sugar, divided
- 3 tablespoons canola oil
- 2 tablespoons dark brown sugar
- 1 teaspoon grated orange zest
- 1 teaspoon vanilla extract
- 2/3 cup all-purpose flour
- 1/3 cup white whole wheat flour
- 1 teaspoon baking powder
- 2 teaspoons pumpkin pie spice, divided
- 1/4 teaspoon baking soda
- 1/4 teaspoon salt
- 1 cup shredded carrots
- 1/4 cup dried cranberries
- 1/3 cup chopped walnuts, toasted

## DIRECTIONS

1. Preheat air fryer to 350°. Grease and flour a 6-in. round baking pan. In a large bowl, whisk egg, buttermilk, 1/3 cup sugar, oil, brown sugar, orange zest and vanilla. In another bowl, whisk flours, baking powder, 1 teaspoon pumpkin pie spice, baking soda and salt. Gradually beat into egg mixture. Fold in carrots and dried cranberries. Pour into prepared pan.
2. In a small bowl, combine walnuts, remaining 2 tablespoons sugar and remaining 1 teaspoon pumpkin spice. Sprinkle evenly over batter. Gently place pan in the basket of a large air fryer.
3. Cook until a toothpick inserted in center comes out clean, 35-40 minutes. Cover tightly with foil if top gets too dark. Cool in pan on a wire rack for 10 minutes before removing from pan. Serve warm.

# Air-Fryer General Tso's Cauliflower

**TOTAL TIME: Prep: 25 min. Cook: 20 min. Servings: 4**

## INGREDIENTS

- 1/2 cup all-purpose flour
- 1/2 cup cornstarch
- 1 teaspoon salt
- 1 teaspoon baking powder
- 3/4 cup club soda
- 1 medium head cauliflower, cut into 1-inch florets (about 6 cups)

**SAUCE:**

- 1/4 cup orange juice
- 3 tablespoons sugar
- 3 tablespoons soy sauce
- 3 tablespoons vegetable broth
- 2 tablespoons rice vinegar
- 2 teaspoons sesame oil
- 2 teaspoons cornstarch
- 2 tablespoons canola oil
- 2 to 6 dried pasilla or other hot chiles, chopped
- 3 green onions, white part minced, green part thinly sliced
- 3 garlic cloves, minced
- 1 teaspoon grated fresh gingerroot
- 1/2 teaspoon grated orange zest
- 4 cups hot cooked rice

## DIRECTIONS

1. Preheat air fryer to 400°. Combine flour, cornstarch, salt and baking powder. Stir in club soda just until blended (batter will be thin). Toss florets in batter; transfer to a wire rack set over a baking sheet. Let stand 5 minutes. In batches, place cauliflower on greased tray in air-fryer basket. Cook until golden brown and tender, 10-12 minutes.
2. Meanwhile, whisk together first 6 sauce ingredients; whisk in cornstarch until smooth.
3. In a large saucepan, heat canola oil over medium-high heat. Add chiles; cook and stir until fragrant, 1-2 minutes. Add white part of onions, garlic, ginger and orange zest; cook until fragrant, about 1 minute. Stir orange juice mixture; add to saucepan. Bring to a boil; cook and stir until thickened, 2-4 minutes.
4. Add cauliflower to sauce; toss to coat. Serve with rice; sprinkle with thinly sliced green onions.

# Air-Fryer Rosemary Sausage Meatballs

**TOTAL TIME: Prep: 20 min. Cook: 10 min./batch    Servings: 2**

## INGREDIENTS

- 2 tablespoons olive oil
- 4 garlic cloves, minced
- 1 teaspoon curry powder
- 1 large egg, lightly beaten
- 1 jar (4 ounces) diced pimientos, drained
- 1/4 cup dry bread crumbs
- 1/4 cup minced fresh parsley
- 1 tablespoon minced fresh rosemary
- 2 pounds bulk pork sausage
- Pretzel sticks, optional

## DIRECTIONS

1. Preheat air fryer to 400°. In a small skillet, heat oil over medium heat; saute garlic with curry powder until tender, 1-2 minutes. Cool slightly.
2. In a bowl, combine egg, pimientos, bread crumbs, parsley, rosemary and garlic mixture. Add sausage; mix lightly but thoroughly.
3. Shape into 1-1/4-in. balls. Place in a single layer on tray in air-fryer basket; cook until lightly browned and cooked through, 7-10 minutes. If desired, serve with pretzels.

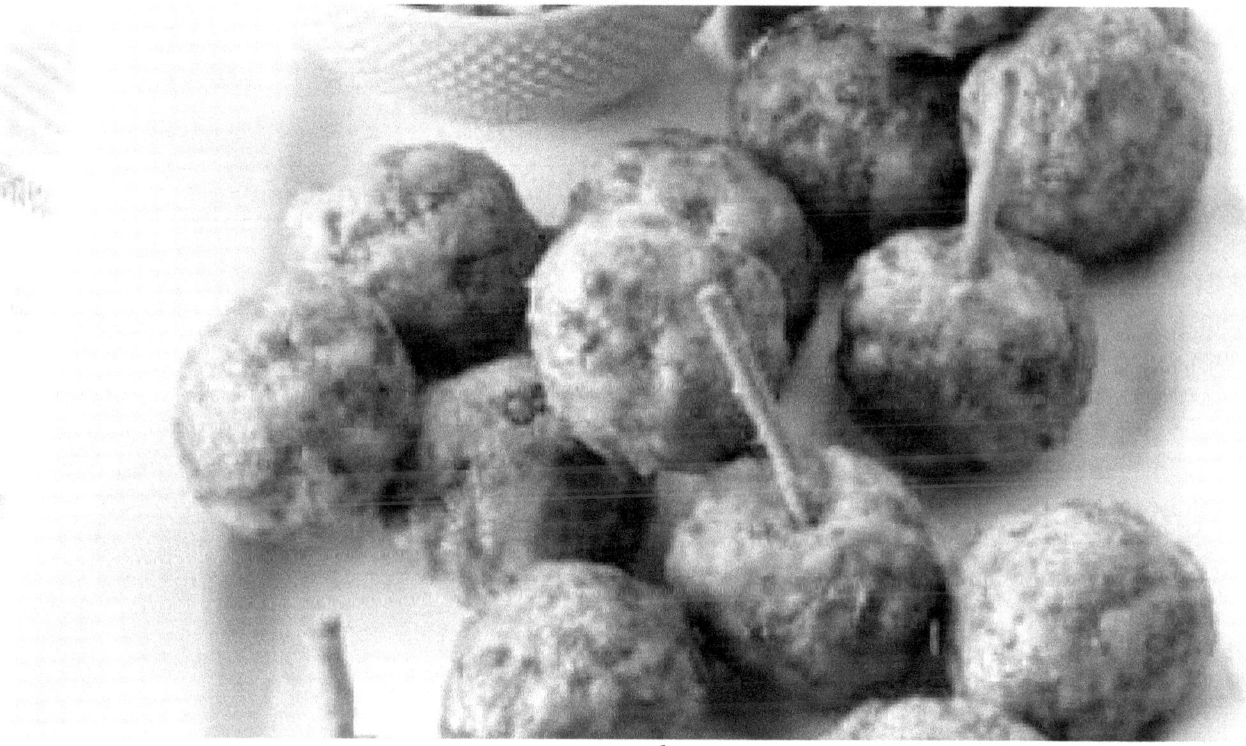

# Air-Fryer Apple Fritters

**TOTAL TIME: Prep: 10 min. Cook: 10 min./batch    Servings: 15**

## INGREDIENTS

- 1-1/2 cups all-purpose flour
- 1/4 cup sugar
- 2 teaspoons baking powder
- 1-1/2 teaspoons ground cinnamon
- 1/2 teaspoon salt
- 2/3 cup 2% milk
- 2 large eggs, room temperature
- 1 tablespoon lemon juice
- 1-1/2 teaspoons vanilla extract, divided
- 2 medium Honeycrisp apples, peeled and chopped
- Cooking spray
- 1/4 cup butter
- 1 cup confectioners' sugar
- 1 tablespoon 2% milk

## DIRECTIONS

1. Preheat air fryer to 410°. In a large bowl, combine flour, sugar, baking powder, cinnamon and salt. Add milk, eggs, lemon juice and 1 teaspoon vanilla extract; stir just until moistened. Fold in apples.

Line air-fryer basket with parchment (cut to fit); spritz with cooking spray. In batches, drop dough by 1/4 cupfuls 2 in. apart onto parchment. Spritz with cooking spray. Cook until golden brown, 5-6 minutes. Turn fritters; continue to air-fry until golden brown, 1-2 minutes.

Melt butter in small saucepan over medium-high heat. Carefully cook until butter starts to brown and foam, about 5 minutes. Remove from heat; cool slightly. Add confectioners' sugar, 1 tablespoon milk and remaining 1/2 teaspoon vanilla extract to browned butter; whisk until smooth. Drizzle over fritters before serving.

◇◇◇◇◇◇◇◇◇◇◇◇◇◇◇◇◇◇◇◇◇◇◇◇◇◇◇◇◇◇◇◇◇◇◇◇◇◇◇◇

# Air-Fryer Keto Meatballs

**TOTAL TIME: Prep: 30 min. Cook: 10 min.    Servings: 4**

## INGREDIENTS

- 1/2 cup grated Parmesan cheese
- 1/2 cup shredded mozzarella cheese
- 1 large egg, lightly beaten
- 2 tablespoons heavy whipping cream
- 1 garlic clove, minced
- 1 pound lean ground beef (90% lean)

**SAUCE:**

- 1 can (8 ounces) tomato sauce with basil, garlic and oregano
- 2 tablespoons prepared pesto
- 1/4 cup heavy whipping cream

## DIRECTIONS

1. Preheat air fryer to 350°. In a large bowl, combine the first 5 ingredients. Add beef; mix lightly but thoroughly. Shape into 1-1/2-in. balls. Place in a single layer on greased tray in air-fryer basket; cook until lightly browned and cooked through, 8-10 minutes.
2. Meanwhile, in a small saucepan, mix sauce ingredients; heat through. Serve with meatballs.

# Air-Fryer Southern-Style Chicken

**TOTAL TIME: Prep:15 min. Cook: 20 min./batch Servings: 6**

**INGREDIENTS**

- 2 cups crushed Ritz crackers (about 50)
- 1 tablespoon minced fresh parsley
- 1 teaspoon garlic salt
- 1 teaspoon paprika
- 1/2 teaspoon pepper
- 1/4 teaspoon ground cumin
- 1/4 teaspoon rubbed sage
- 1 large egg, beaten
- 1 broiler/fryer chicken (3 to 4 pounds), cut up
- Cooking spray

**DIRECTIONS**

1. Preheat air fryer to 375°. In a shallow bowl, mix the first 7 ingredients. Place egg in a separate shallow bowl. Dip chicken in egg, then in cracker mixture, patting to help coating adhere. In batches, place chicken in a single layer on greased tray in air-fryer basket; spritz with cooking spray.
2. Cook 10 minutes. Turn chicken and spritz with cooking spray. Cook until chicken is golden brown and juices run clear, 10-20 minutes longer.

# Air-Fryer Asparagus

**TOTAL TIME: Prep/Total Time: 20 min. Servings: 4**

**INGREDIENTS**

- 1/4 cup mayonnaise
- 4 teaspoons olive oil
- 1-1/2 teaspoons grated lemon zest
- 1 garlic clove, minced
- 1/2 teaspoon pepper
- 1/4 teaspoon seasoned salt
- 1 pound fresh asparagus, trimmed
- 2 tablespoons shredded Parmesan cheese
- Lemon wedges, optional

**DIRECTIONS**

1. Preheat air fryer to 375°. In large bowl, combine the first 6 ingredients. Add asparagus; toss to coat. Working in batches, place in a single layer on greased tray in air-fryer basket.
2. Cook until tender and lightly browned, 4-6 minutes. Transfer to a serving platter; sprinkle with Parmesan cheese. If desired, serve with lemon wedges.

# Air-Fryer Mini Chimichangas

**TOTAL TIME: Prep: 1 hour Cook: 10 min./batch Servings: 14**

## INGREDIENTS

- 1 pound ground beef
- 1 medium onion, chopped
- 1 envelope taco seasoning
- 3/4 cup water
- 3 cups shredded Monterey Jack cheese
- 1 cup sour cream
- 1 can (4 ounces) chopped green chiles, drained
- 14 egg roll wrappers
- 1 large egg white, lightly beaten
- Cooking spray
- Salsa

## DIRECTIONS

1. In a large skillet, cook beef and onion over medium heat until meat is no longer pink; crumble meat; drain. Stir in taco seasoning and water. Bring to a boil. Reduce heat; simmer, uncovered, for 5 minutes, stirring occasionally. Remove from the heat; cool slightly.
2. Preheat air fryer to 375°. In a large bowl, combine cheese, sour cream and chiles. Stir in beef mixture. Place an egg roll wrapper on work surface with a corner facing you. Place 1/3 cup filling in center. Fold bottom one-third of wrapper over filling; fold in sides.
3. Brush top point with egg white; roll up to seal. Repeat with remaining wrappers and filling. (Keep remaining egg roll wrappers covered with waxed paper to keep them from drying out.)
4. In batches, place chimichangas in a single layer on greased tray in air-fryer basket; spritz with cooking spray. Cook until golden brown, 3-4 minutes on each side. Serve warm with salsa and additional sour cream.

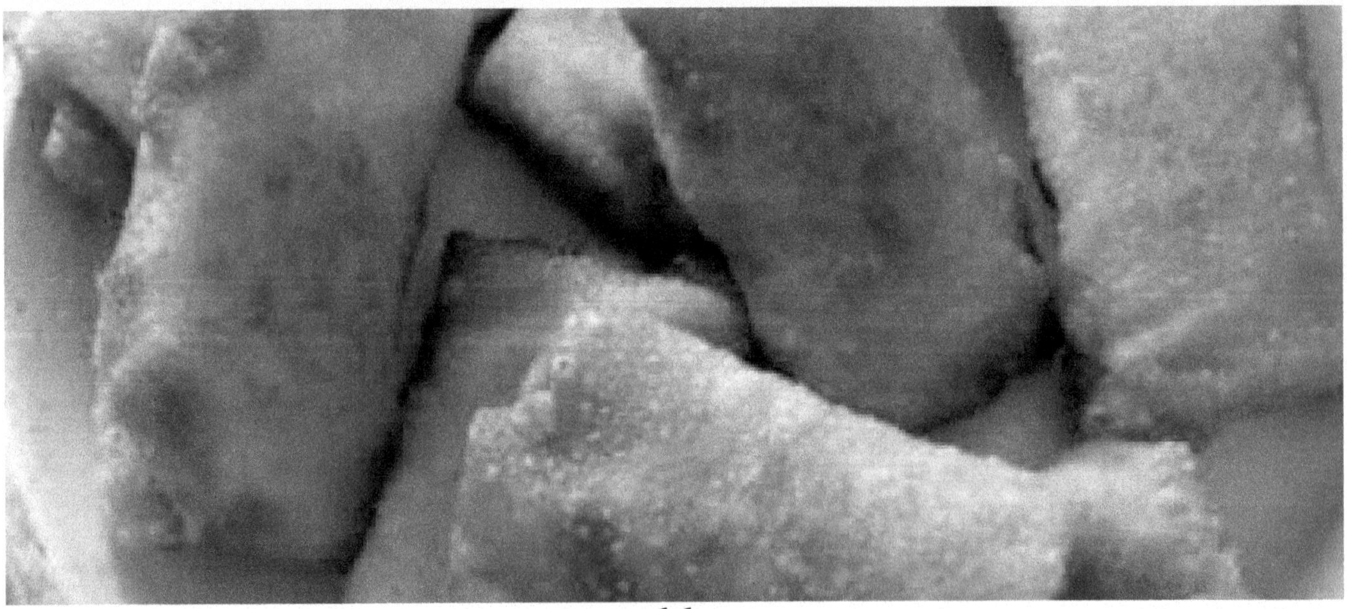

# Cheesy Breakfast Egg Rolls

**TOTAL TIME: Prep: 30 min. Cook: 10 min./batch Servings: 12**

## INGREDIENTS

- 1/2 pound bulk pork sausage
- 1/2 cup shredded sharp cheddar cheese
- 1/2 cup shredded Monterey Jack cheese
- 1 tablespoon chopped green onions
- 4 large eggs
- 1 tablespoon 2% milk
- 1/4 teaspoon salt
- 1/8 teaspoon pepper
- 1 tablespoon butter
- 12 egg roll wrappers
- Cooking spray
- Optional: Maple syrup or salsa

## DIRECTIONS

1. In a small nonstick skillet, cook sausage over medium heat until no longer pink, 4-6 minutes, breaking it into crumbles; drain. Stir in cheeses and green onions; set aside. Wipe skillet clean.
2. In a small bowl, whisk eggs, milk, salt and pepper until blended. In the same skillet, heat butter over medium heat. Pour in egg mixture; cook and stir until eggs are thickened and no liquid egg remains. Stir in sausage mixture.
3. Preheat air fryer to 400°. With 1 corner of an egg roll wrapper facing you, place 1/4 cup filling just below center of wrapper. (Cover remaining wrappers with a damp paper towel until ready to use.) Fold bottom corner over filling; moisten remaining wrapper edges with water. Fold side corners toward center over filling. Roll egg roll up tightly, pressing at tip to seal. Repeat.
4. In batches, arrange egg rolls in a single layer on greased tray in air-fryer basket; spritz with cooking spray. Cook until lightly browned, 3-4 minutes. Turn; spritz with cooking spray. Cook until golden brown and crisp, 3-4 minutes longer. If desired, serve with maple syrup or salsa.

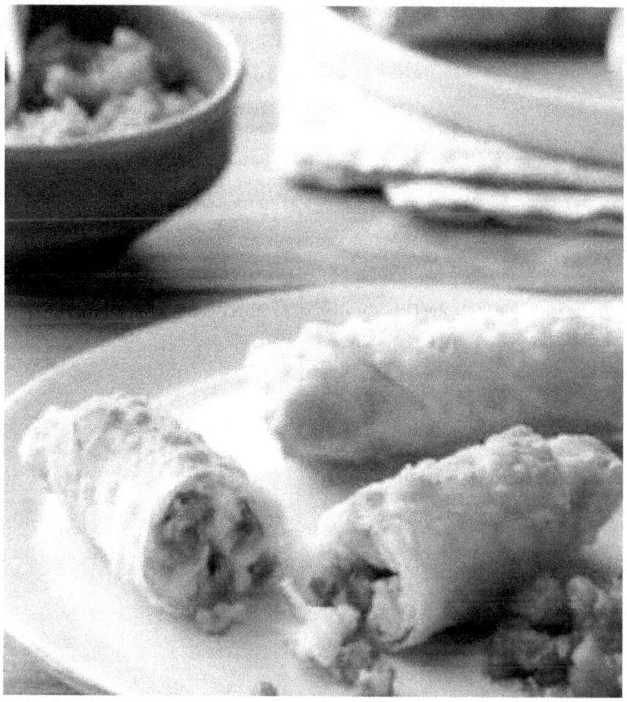

# Air-Fryer Lemon Slice Sugar Cookies

**TOTAL TIME: Prep: 15 min. + chilling Cook: 10 min./ batch + cooling Servings: 2**

## INGREDIENTS

- 1/2 cup unsalted butter, softened
- 1 package (3.4 ounces) instant lemon pudding mix
- 1/2 cup sugar
- 1 large egg, room temperature
- 2 tablespoons 2% milk
- 1-1/2 cups all-purpose flour
- 1 teaspoon baking powder
- 1/4 teaspoon salt

**ICING:**

- 2/3 cup confectioners' sugar
- 2 to 4 teaspoons lemon juice

## DIRECTIONS

1. In a large bowl, cream butter, pudding mix and sugar until light and fluffy, 5-7 minutes. Beat in egg and milk. In another bowl, whisk flour, baking powder and salt; gradually beat into creamed mixture.
2. Divide dough in half. On a lightly floured surface, shape each into a 6-in.-long roll. Wrap and refrigerate 3 hours or until firm.
3. Preheat air fryer to 325°. Unwrap and cut dough crosswise into 1/2-in. slices. In batches, place slices in a single layer on greased tray in air-fryer basket. Cook until edges are light brown, 8-12 minutes. Cool in basket 2 minutes. Remove to wire racks to cool completely.
4. In a small bowl, mix confectioners' sugar and enough lemon juice to reach a drizzling consistency. Drizzle over cookies. Let stand until set.
5. To Make Ahead: Dough can be made 2 days in advance. Wrap and place in a resealable container. Store in the refrigerator.

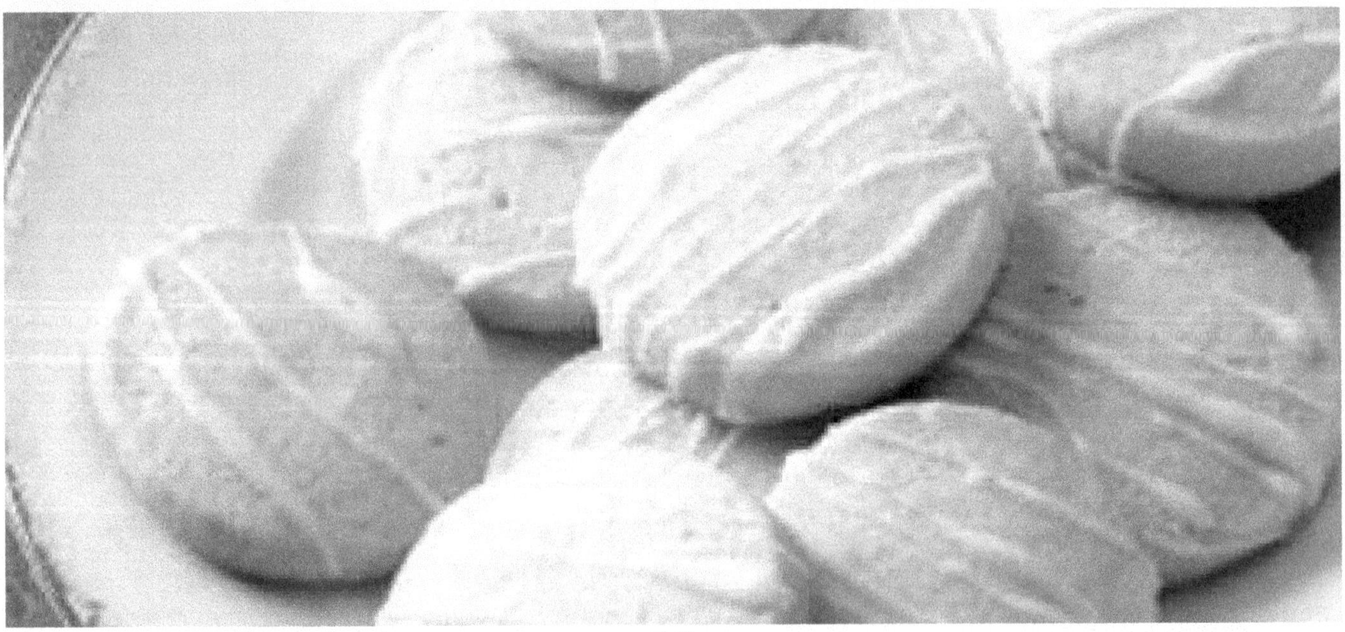

## Air-Fryer Fiesta Chicken Fingers

**TOTAL TIME: Prep: 20 min. Cook: 15 min./batch Servings: 4**

### INGREDIENTS

- 3/4 pound boneless skinless chicken breasts
- 1/2 cup buttermilk
- 1/4 teaspoon pepper
- 1 cup all-purpose flour
- 3 cups corn chips, crushed
- 1 envelope taco seasoning
- Sour cream ranch dip or salsa

### DIRECTIONS

1. Preheat air fryer to 400°. Pound chicken breasts with a meat mallet to 1/2-in. thickness. Cut into 1-in. wide strips.
2. In a shallow bowl, whisk buttermilk and pepper. Place flour in a separate shallow bowl. Mix corn chips and taco seasoning in a third bowl. Dip chicken in flour to coat both sides; shake off excess. Dip in buttermilk mixture, then in corn chip mixture, patting to help coating adhere.
3. In batches, arrange chicken in a single layer on greased tray in air-fryer basket; spritz with cooking spray. Cook until coating is golden brown and chicken is no longer pink, 7-8 minutes on each side. Repeat with remaining chicken. Serve with ranch dip or salsa.

◇◇◇◇◇◇◇◇◇◇◇◇◇◇◇◇◇◇◇◇◇◇◇◇◇◇◇◇◇◇◇◇◇◇◇◇◇◇◇◇

## Air-Fryer Everything Bagel Chicken Strips

**TOTAL TIME: Prep: 10 min. Cook: 15 min./batch Servings: 4**

### INGREDIENTS

- 1 day-old everything bagel, torn
- 1/2 cup panko bread crumbs
- 1/2 cup grated Parmesan cheese
- 1/4 teaspoon crushed red pepper flakes
- 1/4 cup butter, cubed
- 1 pound chicken tenderloins
- 1/2 teaspoon salt

### DIRECTIONS

1. Preheat air fryer to 400°. Pulse torn bagel in a food processor until coarse crumbs form. Place 1/2 cup bagel crumbs in a shallow bowl; toss with panko, cheese and pepper flakes. (Discard or save remaining bagel crumbs for another use.)
2. In a microwave-safe shallow bowl, microwave butter until melted. Sprinkle chicken with salt. Dip in warm butter, then coat with crumb mixture, patting to help adhere. In batches, place chicken in a single layer on greased tray in air-fryer basket.
3. Cook 7 minutes; turn chicken. Continue cooking until coating is golden brown and chicken is no longer pink, 7-8 minutes. Serve immediately.

# Air-Fryer Loaded Pork Burritos

**TOTAL TIME: Prep: 35 min. + marinating Cook: 10 min./batch     Servings: 6**

## INGREDIENTS

- 3/4 cup thawed limeade concentrate
- 1 tablespoon olive oil
- 2 teaspoons salt, divided
- 1-1/2 teaspoons pepper, divided
- 1-1/2 pounds boneless pork loin, cut into thin strips
- 1 cup chopped seeded plum tomatoes
- 1 small green pepper, chopped
- 1 small onion, chopped
- 1/4 cup plus 1/3 cup minced fresh cilantro, divided
- 1 jalapeno pepper, seeded and chopped
- 1 tablespoon lime juice
- 1/4 teaspoon garlic powder
- 1 cup uncooked long grain rice
- Cooking spray
- 3 cups shredded Monterey Jack cheese
- 6 flour tortillas (12 inches), warmed
- 1 can (15 ounces) black beans, rinsed and drained
- 1-1/2 cups sour cream

## DIRECTIONS

1. In a large shallow dish, combine the limeade concentrate, oil, 1 teaspoon salt and 1/2 teaspoon pepper; add pork. Turn to coat; cover and refrigerate at least 20 minutes.
2. For salsa, in a small bowl, combine the tomatoes, green pepper, onion, 1/4 cup cilantro, jalapeno, lime juice, garlic powder, and remaining salt and pepper. Set aside.
3. Meanwhile, cook rice according to package directions. Stir in remaining cilantro; keep warm.
4. Drain pork, discarding marinade. Preheat air fryer to 350°. In batches, place pork in a single layer on greased tray in air-fryer basket; spritz with cooking spray. Cook until pork is no longer pink, 8-10 minutes, turning halfway through.
5. Sprinkle 1/3 cup cheese off-center on each tortilla. Layer each with 1/4 cup salsa, 1/2 cup rice mixture, 1/4 cup black beans and 1/4 cup sour cream; top with about 1/2 cup pork. Fold sides and ends over filling. Serve with remaining salsa.

## Air-Fryer French Toast Sticks

**TOTAL TIME: Prep: 20 min. + freezing Cook: 10 min.    Servings: 1-1/2**

### INGREDIENTS

- 6 slices day-old Texas toast
- 4 large eggs
- 1 cup 2% milk
- 2 tablespoons sugar
- 1 teaspoon vanilla extract
- 1/4 to 1/2 teaspoon ground cinnamon
- 1 cup crushed cornflakes, optional
- Confectioners' sugar, optional
- Maple syrup

### DIRECTIONS

1. Cut each piece of bread into thirds; place in an ungreased 13x9-in. dish. In a large bowl, whisk eggs, milk, sugar, vanilla and cinnamon. Pour over bread; soak for 2 minutes, turning once. If desired, coat bread with cornflake crumbs on all sides.
2. Place in a greased 15x10x1-in. baking pan. Freeze until firm, about 45 minutes. Transfer to an airtight freezer container and store in the freezer.
3. To use frozen French toast sticks: Preheat air fryer to 350°. Place desired number on greased tray in air-fryer basket. Cook for 3 minutes. Turn; cook until golden brown, 2-3 minutes longer. Sprinkle with confectioners' sugar if desired. Serve with syrup.

## Garlic-Herb Fried Patty Pan Squash

**TOTAL TIME: Prep/Total Time: 25 min.    Servings: 4**

### INGREDIENTS

- 5 cups halved small pattypan squash (about 1-1/4 pounds)
- 1 tablespoon olive oil
- 2 garlic cloves, minced
- 1/2 teaspoon salt
- 1/4 teaspoon dried oregano
- 1/4 teaspoon dried thyme
- 1/4 teaspoon pepper
- 1 tablespoon minced fresh parsley

### DIRECTIONS

1. Preheat air fryer to 375°. Place squash in a large bowl. Mix oil, garlic, salt, oregano, thyme and pepper; drizzle over squash. Toss to coat. Place squash on greased tray in air-fryer basket. Cook until tender, 10-15 minutes, stirring occasionally. Sprinkle with parsley.

# Air-Fryer Quinoa Arancini

**TOTAL TIME: Prep/Total Time: 25 min. Servings: 3**

## INGREDIENTS

- 1 package (9 ounces) ready-to-serve quinoa or 1-3/4 cups cooked quinoa
- 2 large eggs, lightly beaten, divided use
- 1 cup seasoned bread crumbs, divided
- 1/4 cup shredded Parmesan cheese
- 1 tablespoon olive oil
- 2 tablespoons minced fresh basil or 2 teaspoons dried basil
- 1/2 teaspoon garlic powder
- 1/2 teaspoon salt
- 1/8 teaspoon pepper
- 6 cubes part-skim mozzarella cheese (3/4 inch each)
- Cooking spray
- Warmed pasta sauce, optional

## DIRECTIONS

1. Preheat air fryer to 375°. Prepare quinoa according to package directions. Stir in 1 egg, 1/2 cup bread crumbs, Parmesan cheese, oil, basil and seasonings.
2. Divide into 6 portions. Shape each portion around a cheese cube to cover completely, forming a ball.
3. Place remaining egg and 1/2 cup bread crumbs in separate shallow bowls. Dip quinoa balls in egg, then roll in bread crumbs. Place on greased tray in air-fryer basket; spritz with cooking spray. Cook until golden brown, 6-8 minutes. If desired, serve with pasta sauce.

◇◇◇◇◇◇◇◇◇◇◇◇◇◇◇◇◇◇◇◇◇◇◇◇◇◇◇◇◇◇◇◇◇◇◇◇◇◇◇◇

# Air-Fryer Chicken Tenders

**TOTAL TIME: Prep: 25 min. Cook: 15 min./batch Servings: 4**

## INGREDIENTS

- 1/2 cup panko bread crumbs
- 1/2 cup potato sticks, crushed
- 1/2 cup crushed cheese crackers
- 1/4 cup grated Parmesan cheese
- 2 bacon strips, cooked and crumbled
- 2 teaspoons minced fresh chives
- 1/4 cup butter, melted
- 1 tablespoon sour cream
- 1 pound chicken tenderloins
- Additional sour cream and chives

## DIRECTIONS

1. Preheat air fryer to 400°. In a shallow bowl, combine the first 6 ingredients. In another shallow bowl, whisk butter and sour cream. Dip chicken in butter mixture, then in crumb mixture, patting to help coating adhere.
2. In batches, arrange chicken in a single layer on greased tray in air-fryer basket; spritz with cooking spray. Cook until coating is golden brown and chicken is no longer pink, 7-8 minutes on each side. Serve with additional sour cream and chives.

# Air-Fryer Turkey Croquettes

**TOTAL TIME: Prep: 20 min. Cook: 10 min./batch    Servings: 6**

## INGREDIENTS

- 2 cups mashed potatoes (with added milk and butter)
- 1/2 cup grated Parmesan cheese
- 1/2 cup shredded Swiss cheese
- 1 shallot, finely chopped
- 2 teaspoons minced fresh rosemary or 1/2 teaspoon dried rosemary, crushed
- 1 teaspoon minced fresh sage or 1/4 teaspoon dried sage leaves
- 1/2 teaspoon salt
- 1/4 teaspoon pepper
- 3 cups finely chopped cooked turkey
- 1 large egg
- 2 tablespoons water
- 1-1/4 cups panko bread crumbs
- Butter-flavored cooking spray
- Sour cream, optional

## DIRECTIONS

1. 1. Preheat air fryer to 350°. In a large bowl, combine mashed potatoes, cheeses, shallot, rosemary, sage, salt and pepper; stir in turkey. Mix lightly but thoroughly. Shape into twelve 1-in.-thick patties.
2. 2. In a shallow bowl, whisk egg and water. Place bread crumbs in another shallow bowl. Dip croquettes in egg mixture, then in bread crumbs, patting to help coating adhere.
3. 3. Working in batches, place croquettes in a single layer on greased tray in air-fryer basket; spritz with cooking spray. Cook until golden brown, 4-5 minutes. Turn; spritz with cooking spray. Cook until golden brown; 4-5 minutes. If desired, serve with sour cream.

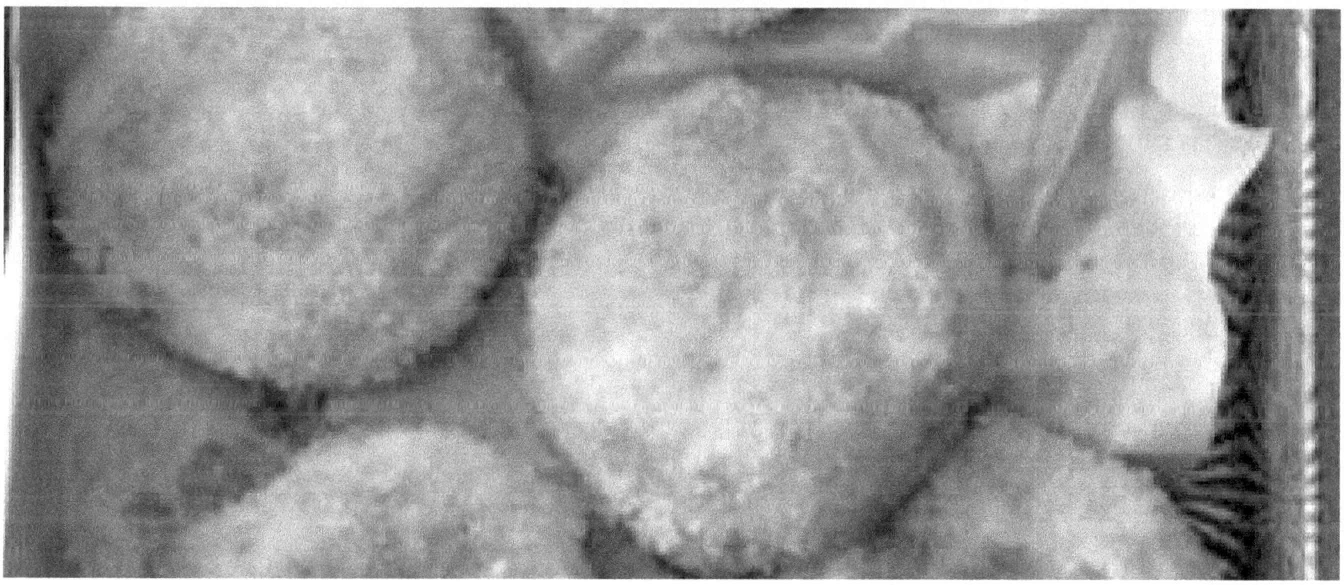

## Air-Fryer Sausage Pizza

**TOTAL TIME: Prep: 30 min. Bake: 10 min./batch Servings: 4**

### INGREDIENTS

- 1 loaf (1 pound) frozen bread dough, thawed
- 1 cup pizza sauce
- 1/2 pound bulk Italian sausage, cooked and drained
- 1-1/3 cups shredded part-skim mozzarella cheese
- 1 small green pepper, sliced into rings
- 1 teaspoon dried oregano
- Crushed red pepper flakes, optional

### DIRECTIONS

1. On a lightly floured surface, roll and stretch dough into four 4-in. circles. Cover; let rest for 10 minutes.
2. Preheat air fryer to 400°. Roll and stretch each dough into a 6-in. circle. Place 1 crust in greased air fryer. Carefully spread with 1/4 cup pizza sauce, 1/3 cup sausage, 1/3 cup cheese, a fourth of the green pepper rings and a pinch of oregano. Cook until crust is golden brown, 6-8 minutes. If desired, sprinkle with red pepper flakes. Repeat with remaining ingredients.

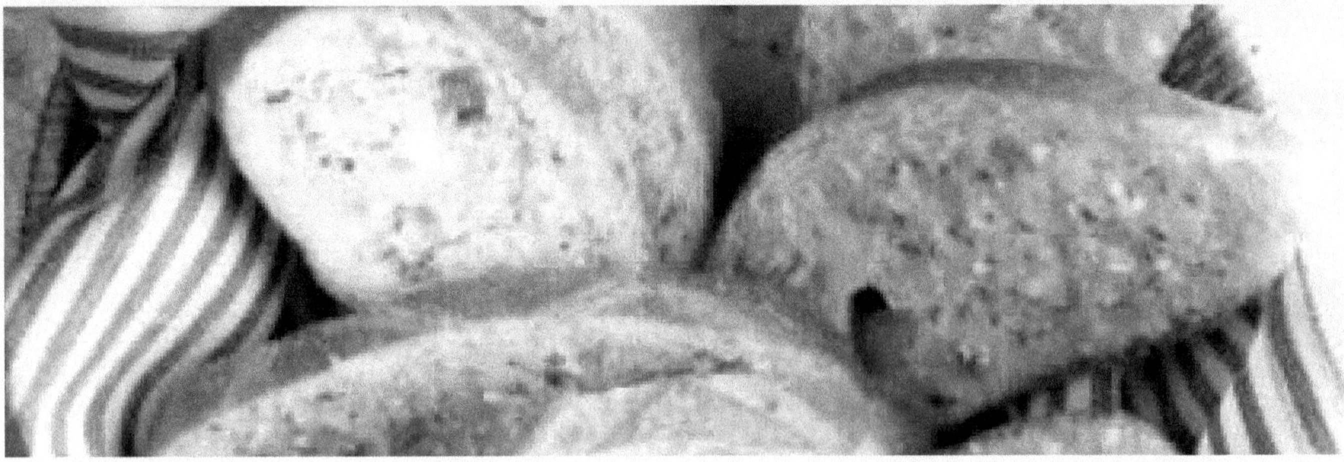

## Air-Fryer Garlic Bread

**TOTAL TIME: Prep/Total Time: 20 min. Servings: 8**

### INGREDIENTS

- 1/4 cup butter, softened
- 3 tablespoons grated Parmesan cheese
- 2 garlic cloves, minced
- 2 teaspoons minced fresh parsley or 1/2 teaspoon dried parsley flakes
- 8 slices ciabatta or French bread

### DIRECTIONS

1. Preheat air fryer to 350°. In a small bowl, combine first 4 ingredients; spread over bread.
2. In batches, arrange bread in a single layer on tray in air-fryer basket. Cook until golden brown, 2-3 minutes. Serve warm.

# Air-Fryer Greek Breadsticks

**TOTAL TIME: Prep: 20 min. Cook: 15 min./batch  Servings: 32**

## INGREDIENTS

- 1/4 cup marinated quartered artichoke hearts, drained
- 2 tablespoons pitted Greek olives
- 1 package (17.3 ounces) frozen puff pastry, thawed
- 1 carton (6-1/2 ounces) spreadable spinach and artichoke cream cheese
- 2 tablespoons grated Parmesan cheese
- 1 large egg
- 1 tablespoon water
- 2 teaspoons sesame seeds
- Refrigerated tzatziki sauce, optional

## DIRECTIONS

1. 1. Preheat air fryer to 325°. Place artichokes and olives in a food processor; cover and pulse until finely chopped. Unfold 1 pastry sheet on a lightly floured surface; spread half the cream cheese over half the pastry. Top with half the artichoke mixture. Sprinkle with half the Parmesan cheese. Fold plain half over filling; press gently to seal.
2. 2. Repeat with remaining pastry, cream cheese, artichoke mixture and Parmesan cheese. Whisk egg and water; brush over tops. Sprinkle with sesame seeds. Cut each rectangle into sixteen 3/4-in.-wide strips. Twist each strip several times.
3. 3. In batches, arrange breadsticks in a single layer on greased tray in air-fryer basket. Cook until golden brown, 12-15 minutes. Serve warm with tzatziki sauce if desired.

◇◇◇◇◇◇◇◇◇◇◇◇◇◇◇◇◇◇◇◇◇◇◇◇◇◇◇◇◇◇◇◇◇◇◇◇◇◇◇◇◇

# Air-Fryer Crumb-Topped Sole

**TOTAL TIME: Prep: 10 min. Cook: 10 min./batch  Servings: 4**

## INGREDIENTS

- 3 tablespoons reduced-fat mayonnaise
- 3 tablespoons grated Parmesan cheese, divided
- 2 teaspoons mustard seed
- 1/4 teaspoon pepper
- 4 sole fillets (6 ounces each)
- 1 cup soft bread crumbs
- 1 green onion, finely chopped
- 1/2 teaspoon ground mustard
- 2 teaspoons butter, melted
- Cooking spray

## DIRECTIONS

1. Preheat air fryer to 375°. Combine mayonnaise, 2 tablespoons cheese, mustard seed and pepper; spread over tops of fillets.
2. Place fish in a single layer on greased tray in air-fryer basket. Cook until fish flakes easily with a fork, 3-5 minutes.
3. Meanwhile, in a small bowl, combine bread crumbs, onion, ground mustard and remaining 1 tablespoon cheese; stir in butter. Spoon over fillets, patting gently to adhere; spritz topping with cooking spray. Cook until golden brown, 2-3 minutes longer. If desired, sprinkle with additional green onions.

# Air-Fryer Beef Wellington Wontons

**TOTAL TIME: Prep: 35 min. Cook: 10 min./batch Servings: 3-1/2**

## INGREDIENTS

- 1/2 pound lean ground beef (90% lean)
- 1 tablespoon butter
- 1 tablespoon olive oil
- 2 garlic cloves, minced
- 1-1/2 teaspoons chopped shallot
- 1 cup each chopped fresh shiitake, baby portobello and white mushrooms
- 1/4 cup dry red wine
- 1 tablespoon minced fresh parsley
- 1/2 teaspoon salt
- 1/4 teaspoon pepper
- 1 package (12 ounces) wonton wrappers
- 1 large egg
- 1 tablespoon water
- Cooking spray

## DIRECTIONS

1. Preheat air fryer to 325°. In a small skillet, cook and crumble beef over medium heat until no longer pink, 4-5 minutes. Transfer to a large bowl. In the same skillet, heat butter and olive oil over medium-high heat. Add garlic and shallot; cook 1 minute. Stir in mushrooms and wine. Cook until mushrooms are tender, 8-10 minutes; add to beef. Stir in parsley, salt and pepper.
2. Place about 2 teaspoons filling in the center of each wonton wrapper. Combine egg and water. Moisten wonton edges with egg mixture; fold opposite corners over filling and press to seal.
3. In batches, arrange wontons in a single layer on greased tray in air-fryer basket; spritz with cooking spray. Cook until lightly browned, 4-5 minutes. Turn; spritz with cooking spray. Cook until golden brown and crisp, 4-5 minutes longer. Serve warm.

◇◇◇◇◇◇◇◇◇◇◇◇◇◇◇◇◇◇◇◇◇◇◇◇◇◇◇◇◇◇◇◇◇◇◇◇◇◇◇◇◇◇◇◇

# Air-Fryer Chickpea Fritters with Sweet-Spicy Sauce

**TOTAL TIME: Prep: 20 min. Cook: 5 min./batch Servings: 2**

## INGREDIENTS

- 1 cup plain yogurt
- 2 tablespoons sugar
- 1 tablespoon honey
- 1/2 teaspoon salt
- 1/2 teaspoon pepper
- 1/2 teaspoon crushed red pepper flakes

**FRITTERS:**

- 1 can (15 ounces) chickpeas or garbanzo beans, rinsed and drained
- 1 teaspoon ground cumin
- 1/2 teaspoon salt
- 1/2 teaspoon garlic powder
- 1/2 teaspoon ground ginger
- 1 large egg
- 1/2 teaspoon baking soda
- 1/2 cup chopped fresh cilantro
- 2 green onions, thinly sliced

## DIRECTIONS

1. Preheat air fryer to 400°. In a small bowl, combine the first 6 ingredients; refrigerate until serving.
2. Place chickpeas and seasonings in a food processor; process until finely ground. Add egg and baking soda; pulse until blended. Transfer to a bowl; stir in cilantro and green onions.
3. In batches, drop bean mixture by rounded tablespoonfuls onto greased tray in air-fryer basket. Cook until lightly browned, 5-6 minutes. Serve with sauce.

# Air-Fryer Nacho Hot Dogs

**TOTAL TIME: Prep: 20 min. Cook: 15 min. Servings: 6**

## INGREDIENTS

- 6 hot dogs
- 3 cheddar cheese sticks, halved lengthwise
- 1-1/4 cups self-rising flour
- 1 cup plain Greek yogurt
- 1/4 cup salsa
- 1/4 teaspoon chili powder
- 3 tablespoons chopped seeded jalapeno pepper
- 1 cup crushed nacho-flavored tortilla chips, divided
- Guacamole and sour cream, optional

## DIRECTIONS

1. Cut a slit down the length of each hot dog without cutting through; insert a halved cheese stick into the slit. Set aside.
2. Preheat air fryer to 350°. In a large bowl, stir together flour, yogurt, salsa, chili powder, jalapenos and 1/4 cup crushed tortilla chips to form a soft dough. Place dough on a lightly floured surface; divide into 6 pieces. Roll dough into 15-inch long strips; wrap one strip around cheese-stuffed hot dog. Repeat with remaining dough and hot dogs. Spray dogs with cooking spray and gently roll in remaining crushed chips. Spray air fryer basket with cooking spray, and place dogs in basket without touching, leaving room to expand.
3. In batches, cook until dough is slightly browned and cheese starts to melt, 8-10 minutes. If desired, serve with additional salsa, sour cream and guacamole.

◇◇◇◇◇◇◇◇◇◇◇◇◇◇◇◇◇◇◇◇◇◇◇◇◇◇◇◇◇◇◇◇◇◇◇◇◇◇◇◇◇◇◇◇

# Air-Fryer Raspberry Balsamic Smoked Pork Chops

**TOTAL TIME: Prep: 15 min. Cook: 15 min./batch Servings: 4**

## INGREDIENTS

- 2 large eggs
- 1/4 cup 2% milk
- 1 cup panko bread crumbs
- 1 cup finely chopped pecans
- 4 smoked bone-in pork chops (7-1/2 ounces each)
- 1/4 cup all-purpose flour
- Cooking spray
- 1/3 cup balsamic vinegar
- 2 tablespoons brown sugar
- 2 tablespoons seedless raspberry jam
- 1 tablespoon thawed frozen orange juice concentrate

## DIRECTIONS

1. Preheat air fryer to 400°. In a shallow bowl, whisk together eggs and milk. In another shallow bowl, toss bread crumbs with pecans.
2. Coat pork chops with flour; shake off excess. Dip in egg mixture, then in crumb mixture, patting to help adhere. In batches, place chops in single layer on greased tray in air-fryer basket; spritz with cooking spray.
3. Cook until golden brown and a thermometer inserted in pork reads 145°, 12-15 minutes, turning halfway through cooking and spritzing with additional cooking spray. Meanwhile, place remaining ingredients in a small saucepan; bring to a boil. Cook and stir until slightly thickened, 6-8 minutes. Serve with chops.

# Air-Fryer Pork Chops

**TOTAL TIME: Prep: 10 min. Cook: 15 min. Servings: 4**

## INGREDIENTS

- 1/3 cup almond flour
- 1/4 cup grated Parmesan cheese
- 1 teaspoon garlic powder
- 1 teaspoon Creole seasoning
- 1 teaspoon paprika
- 4 boneless pork loin chops (6 ounces each)
- Cooking spray

## DIRECTIONS

1. Preheat air fryer to 375°. In a shallow bowl, toss almond flour, cheese, garlic powder, Creole seasoning and paprika. Coat pork chops with flour mixture; shake off excess. Working in batches as needed, place chops in single layer on greased tray in air-fryer basket; spritz with cooking spray.
2. Cook until golden brown, 12-15 minutes or until a thermometer reads 145°, turning halfway through cooking and spritzing with additional cooking spray. Remove and keep warm. Repeat with remaining chops.

# Air-Fryer Crispy Sriracha Spring Rolls

**TOTAL TIME: Prep: 50 min. Cook: 10 min./batch Servings: 2**

## INGREDIENTS

- 3 cups coleslaw mix (about 7 ounces)
- 3 green onions, chopped
- 1 tablespoon soy sauce
- 1 teaspoon sesame oil
- 1 pound boneless skinless chicken breasts
- 1 teaspoon seasoned salt
- 2 packages (8 ounces each) cream cheese, softened
- 2 tablespoons Sriracha chili sauce
- 24 spring roll wrappers
- Cooking spray
- Optional: Sweet chili sauce and additional green onions

## DIRECTIONS

1. Preheat air fryer to 360°. Toss coleslaw mix, green onions, soy sauce and sesame oil; let stand while cooking chicken. Place chicken in a single layer on greased tray in air-fryer basket. Cook until a thermometer inserted in chicken reads 165°, 18-20 minutes. Remove chicken; cool slightly. Finely chop chicken; toss with seasoned salt.
2. Increase air-fryer temperature to 400°. In a large bowl, mix cream cheese and Sriracha chili sauce; stir in chicken and coleslaw mixture. With 1 corner of a spring roll wrapper facing you, place about 2 tablespoons filling just below center of wrapper. (Cover remaining wrappers with a damp paper towel until ready to use.) Fold bottom corner over filling; moisten remaining edges with water. Fold side corners toward center over filling; roll up tightly, pressing tip to seal. Repeat.
3. In batches, arrange spring rolls in a single layer on greased tray in air-fryer basket; spritz with cooking spray. Cook until lightly browned, 5-6 minutes. Turn; spritz with cooking spray. Cook until golden brown and crisp, 5-6 minutes longer. If desired, serve with sweet chili sauce and sprinkle with green onions.

# Air-Fryer Shrimp Po'Boys

**TOTAL TIME: Prep: 35 min. Cook: 10 min./batch Servings: 4**

## INGREDIENTS

- 1/2 cup mayonnaise
- 1 tablespoon Creole mustard
- 1 tablespoon chopped cornichons or dill pickles
- 1 tablespoon minced shallot
- 1-1/2 teaspoons lemon juice
- 1/8 teaspoon cayenne pepper

**COCONUT SHRIMP:**

- 1 cup all-purpose flour
- 1 teaspoon herbes de Provence
- 1/2 teaspoon sea salt
- 1/2 teaspoon garlic powder
- 1/2 teaspoon pepper
- 1/4 teaspoon cayenne pepper
- 1 large egg
- 1/2 cup 2% milk
- 1 teaspoon hot pepper sauce
- 2 cups sweetened shredded coconut
- 1 pound uncooked shrimp (26-30 per pound), peeled and deveined
- Cooking spray
- 4 hoagie buns, split
- 2 cups shredded lettuce
- 1 medium tomato, thinly sliced

## DIRECTIONS

1. For remoulade, in a small bowl, combine the first 6 ingredients. Refrigerate, covered, until serving.
2. Preheat air fryer to 375°. In a shallow bowl, mix flour, herbes de Provence, sea salt, garlic powder, pepper and cayenne. In a separate shallow bowl, whisk egg, milk and hot pepper sauce. Place coconut in a third shallow bowl. Dip shrimp in flour to coat both sides; shake off excess. Dip in egg mixture, then in coconut, patting to help adhere.
3. In batches, arrange shrimp in a single layer on greased tray in air-fryer basket; spritz with cooking spray. Cook until coconut is lightly browned and shrimp turn pink, 3-4 minutes on each side.
4. Spread cut side of buns with remoulade. Top with shrimp, lettuce and tomato.

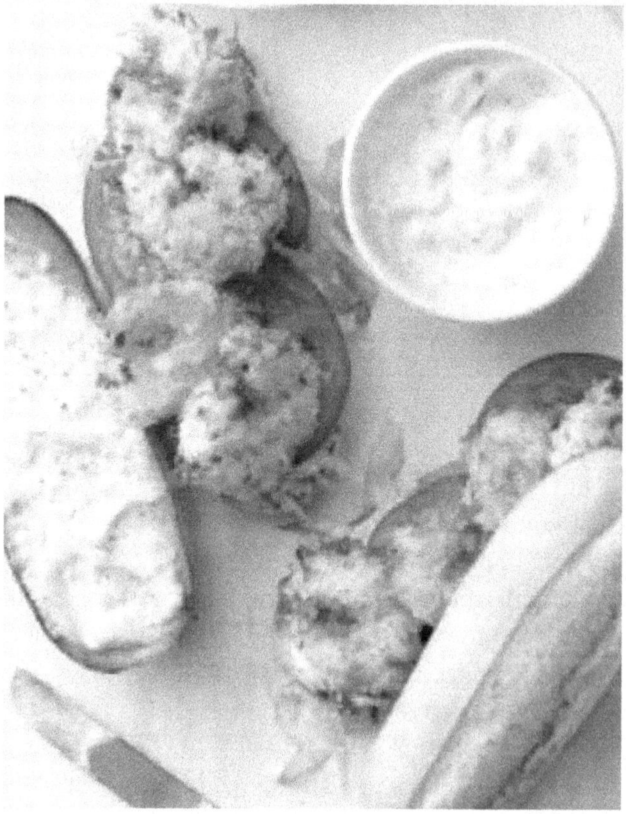

# Air-Fryer S'mores Crescent Rolls

**TOTAL TIME: Prep: 15 min. Cook: 10 min./batch Servings: 8**

## INGREDIENTS

- 1 tube (8 ounces) refrigerated crescent rolls
- 1/4 cup Nutella, divided
- 2 whole graham crackers, broken up
- 2 tablespoons milk chocolate chips
- 2/3 cup miniature marshmallows

## DIRECTIONS

1. Preheat air fryer to 300°. Unroll crescent dough; separate into 8 triangles. Place 1 teaspoon Nutella at the wide end of each triangle. Sprinkle with graham crackers, chocolate chips and marshmallows; roll up.
2. In batches, arrange rolls, point side down, in a single layer on greased tray in air-fryer basket. Curve to form crescents. Cook until golden brown, 8-10 minutes. In a microwave, warm remaining Nutella to reach a drizzling consistency; spoon over rolls. Serve warm.

◇◇◇◇◇◇◇◇◇◇◇◇◇◇◇◇◇◇◇◇◇◇◇◇◇◇◇◇◇◇◇◇◇◇◇◇◇◇◇◇◇◇◇◇◇◇◇◇

# Air-Fryer Papas Rellenas

**TOTAL TIME: Prep: 45 min. Cook: 15 min./batch Servings: 2-1/2**

## INGREDIENTS

- 2-1/2 pounds potatoes (about 8 medium), peeled and cut into wedges
- 1 pound lean ground beef (90% lean)
- 1 small green pepper, finely chopped
- 1 small onion, finely chopped
- 1/2 cup tomato sauce
- 1/2 cup sliced green olives with pimientos
- 1/2 cup raisins
- 1-1/4 teaspoons salt, divided
- 1-1/4 teaspoons pepper, divided
- 1/2 teaspoon paprika
- 1 teaspoon garlic powder
- 2 large eggs, lightly beaten
- 1 cup seasoned bread crumbs
- Cooking spray

## DIRECTIONS

1. Place potatoes in a large saucepan and cover with water. Bring to a boil. Reduce heat; cover and cook until tender, 15-20 minutes.
2. Meanwhile, in a large skillet, cook beef, green pepper and onion over medium heat until meat is no longer pink; drain. Stir in tomato sauce, olives, raisins, 1/4 teaspoon salt, 1/4 teaspoon pepper and paprika; heat through.
3. Drain potatoes; mash with garlic powder and remaining 1 teaspoon salt and pepper. Shape 2 tablespoons potatoes into a patty; place a heaping tablespoon of filling in the center. Shape potatoes around filling, forming a ball. Repeat.
4. Place eggs and bread crumbs in separate shallow bowls. Dip potato balls in eggs, then roll in bread crumbs. Preheat air fryer to 400°. In batches, place in single layer on greased tray in air-fryer basket; spritz with cooking spray. Cook until golden brown, 14-16 minutes.

## Air-Fryer French Toast Cups with Raspberries

**TOTAL TIME: Prep: 20 min. + chilling Cook: 20 min. Servings: 2**

### INGREDIENTS

- 2 slices Italian bread, cut into 1/2-inch cubes
- 1/2 cup fresh or frozen raspberries
- 2 ounces cream cheese, cut into 1/2-inch cubes
- 2 large eggs
- 1/2 cup 2% milk
- 1 tablespoon maple syrup

**RASPBERRY SYRUP:**

- 2 teaspoons cornstarch
- 1/3 cup water
- 2 cups fresh or frozen raspberries, divided
- 1 tablespoon lemon juice
- 1 tablespoon maple syrup
- 1/2 teaspoon grated lemon zest
- Ground cinnamon, optional

### DIRECTIONS

1. Divide half the bread cubes between 2 greased 8-oz. custard cups. Sprinkle with raspberries and cream cheese. Top with remaining bread. In a small bowl, whisk eggs, milk and syrup; pour over bread. Cover and refrigerate for at least 1 hour.
2. Preheat air fryer to 325°. Place custard cups on tray in air-fryer basket. Cook until golden brown and puffed, 12-15 minutes.
3. Meanwhile, in a small saucepan, combine cornstarch and water until smooth. Add 1-1/2 cups raspberries, lemon juice, syrup and lemon zest. Bring to a boil; reduce heat. Cook and stir until thickened, about 2 minutes. Strain and discard seeds; cool slightly.
4. Gently stir remaining 1/2 cup berries into syrup. If desired, sprinkle French toast cups with cinnamon; serve with syrup.

◇◇◇◇◇◇◇◇◇◇◇◇◇◇◇◇◇◇◇◇◇◇◇◇◇◇◇◇◇◇◇◇◇◇◇◇◇◇◇◇

## Air Fryer Ham and Cheese Turnovers

**TOTAL TIME: Prep: 20 min. Cook: 10 min./batch Servings: 4**

### INGREDIENTS

- 1 tube (13.8 ounces) refrigerated pizza crust
- 1/4 pound thinly sliced black forest deli ham
- 1 medium pear, thinly sliced and divided
- 1/4 cup chopped walnuts, toasted
- 2 tablespoons crumbled blue cheese

### DIRECTIONS

1. Preheat air fryer to 400°. On a lightly floured surface, unroll pizza crust into a 12-in. square. Cut into 4 squares. Layer ham, half of pear slices, walnuts and blue cheese diagonally over half of each square to within 1/2 in. of edges. Fold 1 corner over filling to the opposite corner, forming a triangle; press edges with a fork to seal.
2. In batches, arrange turnovers in a single layer on greased tray in air-fryer basket; spritz with cooking spray. Cook until golden brown, 4-6 minutes on each side. Garnish with remaining pear slices.

# Air-Fryer Pork Schnitzel

**TOTAL TIME: Prep: 20 min. Cook: 10 min.  Servings: 4**

## INGREDIENTS

- 1/4 cup all-purpose flour
- 1 teaspoon seasoned salt
- 1/4 teaspoon pepper
- 1 large egg
- 2 tablespoons 2% milk
- 3/4 cup dry bread crumbs
- 1 teaspoon paprika
- 4 pork sirloin cutlets (4 ounces each)
- Cooking spray

**DILL SAUCE:**

- 1 tablespoon all-purpose flour
- 3/4 cup chicken broth
- 1/2 cup sour cream
- 1/4 teaspoon dill weed

## DIRECTIONS

1. Preheat air fryer to 375°. In a shallow bowl, mix flour, seasoned salt and pepper. In a second shallow bowl, whisk egg and milk until blended. In a third bowl, mix bread crumbs and paprika.
2. Pound pork cutlets with a meat mallet to 1/4-in. thickness. Dip cutlets in flour mixture to coat both sides; shake off excess. Dip in egg mixture, then in crumb mixture, patting to help coating adhere.
3. Place pork in a single layer on greased tray in air-fryer basket; spritz with cooking spray. Cook until golden brown, 4-5 minutes. Turn; spritz with cooking spray. Cook until golden brown, 4-5 minutes longer. Remove to a serving plate; keep warm.
4. Meanwhile, in a small saucepan, whisk flour and broth until smooth. Bring to a boil, stirring constantly; cook and stir 2 minutes or until thickened. Reduce heat to low. Stir in sour cream and dill; heat through (do not boil). Serve with pork.

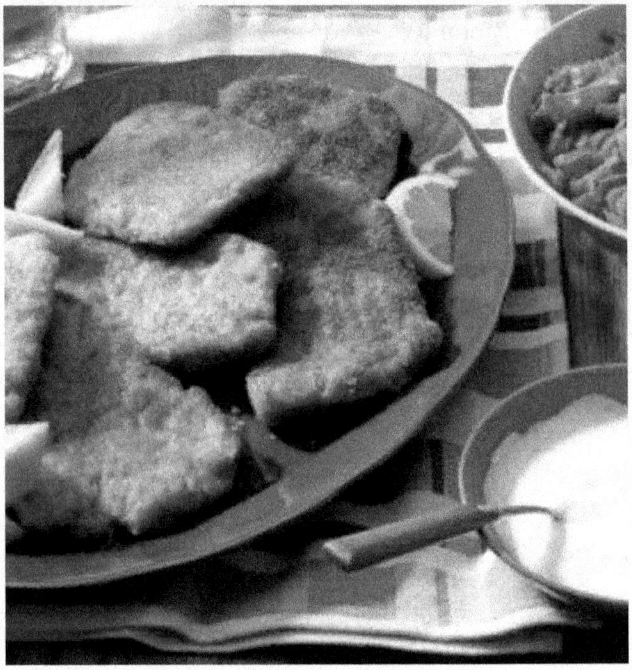

## Air-Fryer Green Tomato Stacks

**TOTAL TIME: Prep: 20 min. Cook: 15 min./batch Servings: 8**

### INGREDIENTS

- 1/4 cup fat-free mayonnaise
- 1/4 teaspoon grated lime zest
- 2 tablespoons lime juice
- 1 teaspoon minced fresh thyme or 1/4 teaspoon dried thyme
- 1/2 teaspoon pepper, divided
- 1/4 cup all-purpose flour
- 2 large egg whites, lightly beaten
- 3/4 cup cornmeal
- 1/4 teaspoon salt
- 2 medium green tomatoes
- 2 medium red tomatoes
- Cooking spray
- 8 slices Canadian bacon, warmed

### DIRECTIONS

1. Preheat air fryer to 375°. Mix mayonnaise, lime zest and juice, thyme and 1/4 teaspoon pepper; refrigerate until serving. Place flour in a shallow bowl; place egg whites in a separate shallow bowl. In a third bowl, mix cornmeal, salt and remaining 1/4 teaspoon pepper.
2. Cut each tomato crosswise into 4 slices. Lightly coat each slice in flour; shake off excess. Dip in egg whites, then in cornmeal mixture.
3. In batches, place tomatoes on greased tray in air-fryer basket; spritz with cooking spray. Cook until golden brown, 4-6 minutes. Turn; spritz with cooking spray. Cook until golden brown, 4-6 minutes longer.
4. For each serving, stack 1 slice each green tomato, bacon and red tomato. Serve with sauce.

◇◇◇◇◇◇◇◇◇◇◇◇◇◇◇◇◇◇◇◇◇◇◇◇◇◇◇◇◇◇◇◇◇◇◇◇◇◇◇◇◇

## Air-Fryer Pretzel-Crusted Catfish

**TOTAL TIME: Prep: 15 min. Cook: 10 min./batch Servings: 4**

### INGREDIENTS

- 4 catfish fillets (6 ounces each)
- 1/2 teaspoon salt
- 1/2 teaspoon pepper
- 2 large eggs
- 1/3 cup Dijon mustard
- 2 tablespoons 2% milk
- 1/2 cup all-purpose flour
- 4 cups honey mustard miniature pretzels, coarsely crushed
- Cooking spray
- Lemon slices, optional

### DIRECTIONS

1. 1. Preheat air fryer to 325°. Sprinkle catfish with salt and pepper. Whisk eggs, mustard and milk in a shallow bowl. Place flour and pretzels in separate shallow bowls. Coat fillets with flour, then dip in egg mixture and coat with pretzels.
2. 2. In batches, place fillets in a single layer on greased tray in air-fryer basket; spritz with cooking spray. Cook until fish flakes easily with a fork, 10-12 minutes. If desired, serve with lemon slices.

# Air-Fryer Bread Pudding

**TOTAL TIME: Prep: 15 min. + standing Cook: 15 min. Servings: 2**

## INGREDIENTS

- 2 ounces semisweet chocolate, chopped
- 1/2 cup half-and-half cream
- 2/3 cup sugar
- 1/2 cup 2% milk
- 1 large egg, room temperature
- 1 teaspoon vanilla extract
- 1/4 teaspoon salt
- 4 slices day-old bread, crusts removed and cut into cubes (about 3 cups)
- Optional toppings: Confectioners' sugar and whipped cream

## DIRECTIONS

1. In a small microwave-safe bowl, melt chocolate; stir until smooth. Stir in cream.
2. In a large bowl, whisk sugar, milk, egg, vanilla and salt. Stir in chocolate mixture. Add bread cubes and toss to coat. Let stand 15 minutes.
3. Preheat air fryer to 325°. Spoon bread mixture into 2 greased 8-oz. ramekins. Place on tray in air-fryer basket. Cook until a knife inserted in the center comes out clean, 12-15 minutes.
4. If desired, top with confectioners' sugar and whipped cream.

◇◇◇◇◇◇◇◇◇◇◇◇◇◇◇◇◇◇◇◇◇◇◇◇◇◇◇◇◇◇◇◇◇◇◇◇◇◇◇◇◇

# Air-Fryer Crispy Curry Drumsticks

**TOTAL TIME: Prep: 35 min. Cook: 15 min./batch Servings: 4**

## INGREDIENTS

- 1 pound chicken drumsticks
- 3/4 teaspoon salt, divided
- 2 tablespoons olive oil
- 2 teaspoons curry powder
- 1/2 teaspoon onion salt
- 1/2 teaspoon garlic powder
- Minced fresh cilantro, optional

## DIRECTIONS

1. Place chicken in a large bowl; add 1/2 teaspoon salt and enough water to cover. Let stand 15 minutes at room temperature. Drain and pat dry.
2. Preheat air fryer to 375°. In another bowl, mix oil, curry powder, onion salt, garlic powder and remaining 1/4 teaspoon salt; add chicken and toss to coat. In batches, place chicken in a single layer on tray in air-fryer basket. Cook until a thermometer inserted in chicken reads 170°-175°, 15-17 minutes, turning halfway through. If desired, sprinkle with cilantro.

## Air-Fryer Mini Nutella Doughnut Holes

**TOTAL TIME: Prep: 30 min. Cook: 10 min./batch Servings: 32**

### INGREDIENTS

- 1 large egg
- 1 tablespoon water
- 1 tube (16.3 ounces) large refrigerated flaky biscuits (8 count)
- 2/3 cup Nutella
- Confectioners' sugar

### DIRECTIONS

1. Preheat air fryer to 300°. Whisk egg with water. On a lightly floured surface, roll each biscuit into a 6-in. circle; cut each into 4 wedges. Brush lightly with egg mixture; top each wedge with 1 teaspoon Nutella. Bring up corners over filling; pinch edges firmly to seal.
2. In batches, arrange wedges in a single layer on ungreased tray in air-fryer basket. Cook until golden brown, 8-10 minutes, turning once. Dust with confectioners' sugar; serve warm.

◇◇◇◇◇◇◇◇◇◇◇◇◇◇◇◇◇◇◇◇◇◇◇◇◇◇◇◇◇◇◇◇◇◇◇◇◇◇◇◇◇◇

## Air-Fryer Ground Beef Wellington

**TOTAL TIME: Prep: 30 min. Cook: 20 min. Servings: 2**

### INGREDIENTS

- 1 tablespoon butter
- 1/2 cup chopped fresh mushrooms
- 2 teaspoons all-purpose flour
- 1/4 teaspoon pepper, divided
- 1/2 cup half-and-half cream
- 1 large egg yolk
- 2 tablespoons finely chopped onion
- 1/4 teaspoon salt
- 1/2 pound ground beef
- 1 tube (4 ounces) refrigerated crescent rolls
- 1 large egg, lightly beaten, optional
- 1 teaspoon dried parsley flakes

### DIRECTIONS

1. Preheat air fryer to 300°. In a saucepan, heat butter over medium-high heat. Add mushrooms; cook and stir until tender, 5-6 minutes. Stir in flour and 1/8 teaspoon pepper until blended. Gradually add cream. Bring to a boil; cook and stir for 2 minutes or until thickened. Remove from the heat and set aside.
2. In a bowl, combine egg yolk, onion, 2 tablespoons mushroom sauce, salt and remaining 1/8 teaspoon pepper. Crumble beef over mixture and mix well. Shape into 2 loaves. Unroll crescent dough and separate into 2 rectangles; press perforations to seal. Place meat loaf on each rectangle. Bring edges together and pinch to seal. If desired, brush with beaten egg.
3. Place Wellingtons in a single layer on greased tray in air-fryer basket. Cook until golden brown and a thermometer inserted into meat loaf reads 160°, 18-22 minutes.
4. Meanwhile, warm remaining sauce over low heat; stir in parsley. Serve sauce with Wellingtons.

# Air-Fryer Taquitos

**TOTAL TIME: Prep: 20 min. Cook: 15 min./batch Servings: 10**

## INGREDIENTS

- 2 large eggs
- 1/2 cup dry bread crumbs
- 3 tablespoons taco seasoning
- 1 pound lean ground beef (90% lean)
- 10 corn tortillas (6 inches), warmed
- Cooking spray
- Optional: Salsa and guacamole

## DIRECTIONS

1. Preheat air fryer to 350°. In a large bowl, combine eggs, bread crumbs and taco seasoning. Add beef; mix lightly but thoroughly.

2. Spoon 1/4 cup beef mixture down the center of each tortilla. Roll up tightly and secure with toothpicks. In batches, arrange taquitos in a single layer on greased tray in air-fryer basket; spritz with cooking spray. Cook 6 minutes; turn and cook until meat is cooked through and taquitos are golden brown and crispy, 6-7 minutes longer. Discard toothpicks before serving. If desired, serve with salsa and guacamole.

◇◇◇◇◇◇◇◇◇◇◇◇◇◇◇◇◇◇◇◇◇◇◇◇◇◇◇◇◇◇◇◇◇◇◇◇◇◇◇◇◇◇◇◇◇

# Air-Fryer Nashville Hot Chicken

**TOTAL TIME: Prep: 30 min. + marinating Cook: 10 min./batch Servings: 6**

## INGREDIENTS

- 2 tablespoons dill pickle juice, divided
- 2 tablespoons hot pepper sauce, divided
- 1 teaspoon salt, divided
- 2 pounds chicken tenderloins
- 1 cup all-purpose flour
- 1/2 teaspoon pepper
- 1 large egg
- 1/2 cup buttermilk
- Cooking spray
- 1/2 cup olive oil
- 2 tablespoons cayenne pepper
- 2 tablespoons dark brown sugar
- 1 teaspoon paprika
- 1 teaspoon chili powder
- 1/2 teaspoon garlic powder
- Dill pickle slices

## DIRECTIONS

1. In a bowl or shallow dish, combine 1 tablespoon pickle juice, 1 tablespoon hot sauce and 1/2 teaspoon salt. Add chicken and turn to coat. Refrigerate, covered, at least 1 hour. Drain chicken, discarding any marinade.

2. Preheat air fryer to 375°. In a shallow bowl, mix flour, remaining 1/2 teaspoon salt and the pepper. In another shallow bowl, whisk egg, buttermilk, and the remaining 1 tablespoon pickle juice and 1 tablespoon hot sauce. Dip chicken in flour to coat both sides; shake off excess. Dip in egg mixture, then again in flour mixture.

3. In batches, arrange chicken in a single layer on well-greased tray in air-fryer basket; spritz with cooking spray. Cook until golden brown, 5-6 minutes. Turn; spritz with cooking spray. Cook until golden brown, 5-6 minutes longer.

4. Whisk together the next 6 ingredients; pour over hot chicken and toss to coat. Serve with pickles.

# Air-Fryer Honey Cinnamon Roll-ups

**TOTAL TIME: Prep: 35 min. + cooling Cook: 10 min./batch Servings: 24**

## INGREDIENTS

- 2 cups ground walnuts, toasted
- 1/4 cup sugar
- 2 teaspoons ground cinnamon
- 12 sheets frozen phyllo dough, thawed
- 1/2 cup butter, melted

**SYRUP:**

- 1/2 cup honey
- 1/2 cup sugar
- 1/2 cup water
- 1 tablespoon lemon juice

## DIRECTIONS

1. Preheat air fryer to 325°. Combine walnuts, sugar and cinnamon.
2. Place 1 sheet of phyllo dough on a 15x12-in. piece of waxed paper; brush with butter. Place a second phyllo sheet on top, brushing it with butter. (Keep remaining phyllo covered with a damp towel to prevent it from drying out.) Sprinkle with 1/4 cup walnut mixture. Using waxed paper, roll up tightly jelly-roll style, starting with a long side, removing paper as you roll. Slice roll into 4 smaller rolls. Brush with butter; secure with toothpicks. Repeat with remaining phyllo dough and 1/4 cups of walnut mixture. In batches, place in a single layer on greased tray in air-fryer basket. Cook until light brown, 9-11 minutes. Cool on a wire rack. Discard toothpicks.
3. Meanwhile, in a small saucepan, combine all syrup ingredients. Bring to a boil. Reduce heat; simmer 5 minutes. Cool 10 minutes. Transfer cinnamon rolls to a serving platter; drizzle with syrup. Sprinkle with remaining walnut mixture.

# Air-Fryer Salmon with Maple-Dijon Glaze

**TOTAL TIME: Prep: 10 min. Cook: 15 min. Servings: 4**

## INGREDIENTS

- 3 tablespoons butter
- 3 tablespoons maple syrup
- 1 tablespoon Dijon mustard
- 1 medium lemon (juiced)
- 1 garlic clove, minced
- 1 tablespoon olive oil
- 4 salmon fillets (4 ounces each)
- 1/4 teaspoon salt
- 1/4 teaspoon pepper

## DIRECTIONS

1. Preheat air fryer to 400&deg.
2. In a small saucepan, melt butter over medium-high heat. Add maple syrup, mustard, lemon juice and minced garlic. Reduce heat and simmer until mixture thickens slightly, 2-3 minutes. Remove from heat; set aside.
3. Drizzle olive oil over salmon; sprinkle with salt and pepper. Place fish in a single layer in air-fryer basket. Cook until fish is lightly browned and just beginning to flake easily with a fork, 5-7 minutes. Drizzle with sauce right before serving.

# Air Fryer Sweet and Sour Pineapple Pork

**TOTAL TIME: Prep: 25 min. Cook: 20 min.   Servings: 4**

## INGREDIENTS

- 1 can (8 ounces) unsweetened crushed pineapple, undrained
- 1 cup cider vinegar
- 1/2 cup sugar
- 1/2 cup packed dark brown sugar
- 1/2 cup ketchup
- 2 tablespoons reduced-sodium soy sauce
- 1 tablespoon Dijon mustard
- 1 teaspoon garlic powder
- 2 pork tenderloins (3/4 pound each), halved
- 1/4 teaspoon salt
- 1/4 teaspoon pepper
- Sliced green onions, optional

## DIRECTIONS

1. In a large saucepan, combine the first 8 ingredients. Bring to a boil; reduce heat. Simmer, uncovered, until thickened, 15-20 minutes, stirring occasionally.
2. Preheat air fryer to 350°. Sprinkle pork with salt and pepper. Place pork on greased tray in air-fryer basket. Cook until pork begins to brown around edges, 7-8 minutes. Turn; pour 1/4 cup sauce over pork. Cook until a thermometer inserted into pork reads at least 145°, 10-12 minutes longer. Let pork stand 5 minutes before slicing. Serve with remaining sauce. If desired, top with sliced green onions.

◇◇◇◇◇◇◇◇◇◇◇◇◇◇◇◇◇◇◇◇◇◇◇◇◇◇◇◇◇◇◇◇◇◇◇◇◇◇◇◇

# Air-Fryer Coconut Shrimp and Apricot Sauce

**TOTAL TIME: Prep: 25 min. Cook: 10 min./batch   Servings: 6**

## INGREDIENTS

- 1-1/2 pounds uncooked shrimp (26-30 per pound)
- 1-1/2 cups sweetened shredded coconut
- 1/2 cup panko bread crumbs
- 4 large egg whites
- 3 dashes Louisiana-style hot sauce
- 1/4 teaspoon salt
- 1/4 teaspoon pepper
- 1/2 cup all-purpose flour

## SAUCE:

- 1 cup apricot preserves
- 1 teaspoon cider vinegar
- 1/4 teaspoon crushed red pepper flakes

## DIRECTIONS

1. Preheat air fryer to 375°. Peel and devein shrimp, leaving tails on.
2. In a shallow bowl, toss coconut with bread crumbs. In another shallow bowl, whisk egg whites, hot sauce, salt and pepper. Place flour in a third shallow bowl.
3. Dip shrimp in flour to coat lightly; shake off excess. Dip in egg white mixture, then in coconut mixture, patting to help coating adhere.
4. In batches, place shrimp in a single layer on greased tray in air-fryer basket. Cook 4 minutes. Turn shrimp; cook until coconut is lightly browned and shrimp turn pink, about 4 minutes longer.
5. Meanwhile, combine sauce ingredients in a small saucepan; cook and stir over medium-low heat until preserves are melted. Serve shrimp immediately with sauce.

## Spicy Air-Fryer Chicken Breasts

**TOTAL TIME: Prep: 25 min. + marinating Cook: 20 min./batch Servings: 8**

### INGREDIENTS

- 2 cups buttermilk
- 2 tablespoons Dijon mustard
- 2 teaspoons salt
- 2 teaspoons hot pepper sauce
- 1-1/2 teaspoons garlic powder
- 8 bone-in chicken breast halves, skin removed (8 ounces each)
- 2 cups soft bread crumbs
- 1 cup cornmeal
- 2 tablespoons canola oil
- 1/2 teaspoon poultry seasoning
- 1/2 teaspoon ground mustard
- 1/2 teaspoon paprika
- 1/2 teaspoon cayenne pepper
- 1/4 teaspoon dried oregano
- 1/4 teaspoon dried parsley flakes

### DIRECTIONS

1. Preheat air fryer to 375°. In a large bowl, combine the first 5 ingredients. Add chicken and turn to coat. Refrigerate, covered, 1 hour or overnight.
2. Drain chicken, discarding marinade. Combine remaining ingredients in a shallow dish and stir to combine. Add chicken, 1 piece at a time, and turn to coat. Place in a single layer on greased tray in air-fryer basket. Cook until a thermometer reads 170°, about 20 minutes, turning halfway through cooking. Return all chicken to air fryer and cook to heat through, 2-3 minutes longer.

◇◇◇◇◇◇◇◇◇◇◇◇◇◇◇◇◇◇◇◇◇◇◇◇◇◇◇◇◇◇◇◇◇◇◇◇◇◇◇◇◇◇◇◇

## Air-Fryer Bone-In Pork Chops with Rhubarb

**TOTAL TIME: Prep/Total Time: 20 min. Servings: 2**

### INGREDIENTS

- 2 bone-in pork loin chops (1/2 to 3/4 inch thick)
- 1/4 teaspoon salt
- 1/4 teaspoon pepper
- 2 tablespoons butter
- 1/2 pound fresh or frozen rhubarb, chopped
- 1 tablespoon honey
- 1/8 teaspoon ground cinnamon
- 1-1/2 teaspoons minced fresh parsley

### DIRECTIONS

1. Preheat air fryer to 400°. Sprinkle pork chops with salt and pepper. Place chops in greased air fryer. Cook until a thermometer reads 145°, 4-5 minutes on each side.
2. Meanwhile, in a saucepan, melt butter over medium heat. Add rhubarb, honey and cinnamon; cook until rhubarb is tender, about 5 minutes. Serve sauce over pork chops. Sprinkle with parsley.

# Air-Fryer Green Tomato BLT

**TOTAL TIME: Prep: 20 min. Cook 10 min./batch Servings: 4**

## INGREDIENTS

- 2 medium green tomatoes (about 10 ounces)
- 1/2 teaspoon salt
- 1/4 teaspoon pepper
- 1 large egg, beaten
- 1/4 cup all-purpose flour
- 1 cup panko bread crumbs
- Cooking spray
- 1/2 cup reduced-fat mayonnaise
- 2 green onions, finely chopped
- 1 teaspoon snipped fresh dill or 1/4 teaspoon dill weed
- 8 slices whole wheat bread, toasted
- 8 cooked center-cut bacon strips
- 4 Bibb or Boston lettuce leaves

## DIRECTIONS

1. Preheat air fryer to 350°. Cut each tomato crosswise into 4 slices. Sprinkle with salt and pepper. Place egg, flour and bread crumbs in separate shallow bowls. Dip tomato slices in flour, shaking off excess, then dip into egg, and finally into bread crumb mixture, patting to help adhere.
2. In batches, arrange tomato slices in a single layer on greased tray in air-fryer basket; spritz with cooking spray. Cook until golden brown, 4-6 minutes. Turn; spritz with cooking spray. Cook until golden brown, 4-6 minutes longer.
3. Meanwhile, mix mayonnaise, green onions and dill. Layer each of 4 slices of bread with 2 bacon strips, 1 lettuce leaf and 2 tomato slices. Spread mayonnaise mixture over remaining slices of bread; place over top. Serve immediately.

◇◇◇◇◇◇◇◇◇◇◇◇◇◇◇◇◇◇◇◇◇◇◇◇◇◇◇◇◇◇◇◇◇◇◇◇◇◇◇◇

# Air-Fryer Roasted Green Beans

**TOTAL TIME: Prep: 15 min. Cook: 20 min. Servings: 6**

## INGREDIENTS

- 1 pound fresh green beans, cut into 2 inch pieces
- 1/2 pound sliced fresh mushrooms
- 1 small red onion, halved and thinly sliced
- 2 tablespoons olive oil
- 1 teaspoon Italian seasoning
- 1/4 teaspoon salt
- 1/8 teaspoon pepper

## DIRECTIONS

1. Preheat air fryer to 375°. In a large bowl, combine all ingredients; toss to coat.
2. Arrange vegetables on greased tray in air-fryer basket. Cook until just tender, 8-10 minutes. Toss to redistribute; cook until browned, 8-10 minutes longer.

# Air-Fryer Bourbon Bacon Cinnamon Rolls

**TOTAL TIME: Prep: 25 min. + marinating Cook: 10 min./batch Servings: 8**

**INGREDIENTS**

- 8 bacon strips
- 3/4 cup bourbon
- 1 tube (12.4 ounces) refrigerated cinnamon rolls with icing
- 1/2 cup chopped pecans
- 2 tablespoons maple syrup
- 1 teaspoon minced fresh gingerroot

**DIRECTIONS**

1. Place bacon in a shallow dish; add bourbon. Seal and refrigerate overnight. Remove bacon and pat dry; discard bourbon.
2. In a large skillet, cook bacon in batches over medium heat until nearly crisp but still pliable. Remove to paper towels to drain. Discard all but 1 teaspoon drippings.
3. Preheat air fryer to 350°. Separate dough into 8 rolls, reserving icing packet. Unroll spiral rolls into long strips; pat dough to form 6x1-in. strips. Place 1 bacon strip on each strip of dough, trimming bacon as needed; reroll, forming a spiral. Pinch ends to seal. Repeat with remaining dough. Place 4 rolls on ungreased tray in air-fryer basket; cook 5 minutes. Turn rolls over and cook until golden brown, about 4 minutes.
4. Meanwhile, combine pecans and maple syrup. In another bowl, stir ginger together with contents of icing packet. In same skillet, heat remaining bacon drippings over medium heat. Add pecan mixture; cook, stirring frequently, until lightly toasted, 2-3 minutes.
5. Drizzle half the icing over warm cinnamon rolls; top with half the pecans. Repeat to make a second batch.

◇◇◇◇◇◇◇◇◇◇◇◇◇◇◇◇◇◇◇◇◇◇◇◇◇◇◇◇◇◇◇◇◇◇◇◇◇◇◇◇◇

# Air-Fryer Reuben Calzones

**TOTAL TIME: Prep: 15 min. Cook: 10 min./batch Servings: 4**

**INGREDIENTS**

- 1 tube (13.8 ounces) refrigerated pizza crust
- 4 slices Swiss cheese
- 1 cup sauerkraut, rinsed and well drained
- 1/2 pound sliced cooked corned beef
- Thousand Island salad dressing

**DIRECTIONS**

1. Preheat air fryer to 400°. On a lightly floured surface, unroll pizza crust dough and pat into a 12-in. square. Cut into 4 squares. Layer 1 slice cheese and a fourth of the sauerkraut and corned beef diagonally over half of each square to within 1/2 in. of edges. Fold 1 corner over filling to the opposite corner, forming a triangle; press edges with a fork to seal. Place 2 calzones in a single layer on greased tray in air-fryer basket.
2. Cook until golden brown, 8-12 minutes, flipping halfway through cooking. Serve with salad dressing.

# Air-Fryer Sweet and Sour Pork

**TOTAL TIME: Prep: 25 min. Cook: 20 min. Servings: 2**

**INGREDIENTS**

- 1/2 cup unsweetened crushed pineapple, undrained
- 1/2 cup cider vinegar
- 1/4 cup sugar
- 1/4 cup packed dark brown sugar
- 1/4 cup ketchup
- 1 tablespoon reduced-sodium soy sauce
- 1-1/2 teaspoons Dijon mustard
- 1/2 teaspoon garlic powder
- 1 pork tenderloin (3/4 pound), halved
- 1/8 teaspoon salt
- 1/8 teaspoon pepper
- Cooking spray
- Sliced green onions, optional

**DIRECTIONS**

1. In a small saucepan, combine the first 8 ingredients. Bring to a boil; reduce heat. Simmer, uncovered, until thickened, 6-8 minutes, stirring occasionally.
2. Preheat air fryer to 350°. Sprinkle pork with salt and pepper. Place pork on greased tray in air-fryer basket; spritz with cooking spray. Cook until pork begins to brown around edges, 7-8 minutes. Turn; pour 2 tablespoons sauce over pork. Cook until a thermometer inserted into pork reads at least 145°, 10-12 minutes longer. Let pork stand 5 minutes before slicing. Serve with remaining sauce. If desired, top with sliced green onions.

◇◇◇◇◇◇◇◇◇◇◇◇◇◇◇◇◇◇◇◇◇◇◇◇◇◇◇◇◇◇◇◇◇◇◇◇◇◇◇◇

# Air-Fryer Wasabi Crab Cakes

**TOTAL TIME: Prep: 20 min. Cook: 10 min./batch Servings: 2**

**INGREDIENTS**

- 1 medium sweet red pepper, finely chopped
- 1 celery rib, finely chopped
- 3 green onions, finely chopped
- 2 large egg whites
- 3 tablespoons reduced-fat mayonnaise
- 1/4 teaspoon prepared wasabi
- 1/4 teaspoon salt
- 1/3 cup plus 1/2 cup dry bread crumbs, divided
- 1-1/2 cups lump crabmeat, drained
- Cooking spray

**SAUCE:**

- 1 celery rib, chopped
- 1/3 cup reduced-fat mayonnaise
- 1 green onion, chopped
- 1 tablespoon sweet pickle relish
- 1/2 teaspoon prepared wasabi
- 1/4 teaspoon celery salt

**DIRECTIONS**

1. Preheat air fryer to 375°. Combine first 7 ingredients; add 1/3 cup bread crumbs. Gently fold in crab.
2. Place remaining bread crumbs in a shallow bowl. Drop heaping tablespoons crab mixture into crumbs. Gently coat and shape into 3/4-in.-thick patties. In batches, place patties in a single layer on greased tray in air-fryer basket. Spritz crab cakes with cooking spray. Cook until golden brown, 8-12 minutes, carefully turning halfway through cooking and spritzing with additional cooking spray.
3. Meanwhile, place sauce ingredients in food processor; pulse 2 or 3 times to blend or until desired consistency is reached. Serve crab cakes immediately with dipping sauce.

# Air-Fryer Herb and Cheese-Stuffed Burgers

**TOTAL TIME: Prep: 20 min. Cook: 15 min./batch  Servings: 4**

**INGREDIENTS**

- 2 green onions, thinly sliced
- 2 tablespoons minced fresh parsley
- 4 teaspoons Dijon mustard, divided
- 3 tablespoons dry bread crumbs
- 2 tablespoons ketchup
- 1/2 teaspoon salt
- 1/2 teaspoon dried rosemary, crushed
- 1/4 teaspoon dried sage leaves
- 1 pound lean ground beef (90% lean)
- 2 ounces cheddar cheese, sliced
- 4 hamburger buns, split
- Optional toppings: Lettuce leaves, sliced tomato, mayonnaise and additional ketchup

**DIRECTIONS**

1. Preheat air fryer to 375°. In a small bowl, combine green onions, parsley and 2 teaspoons mustard. In another bowl, mix bread crumbs, ketchup, seasonings and remaining 2 teaspoons mustard. Add beef to bread crumb mixture; mix lightly but thoroughly.
2. Shape mixture into 8 thin patties. Place sliced cheese in center of 4 patties; spoon green onion mixture over cheese. Top with remaining patties, pressing edges together firmly, taking care to seal completely.
3. In batches, place burgers in a single layer on tray in air-fryer basket. Cook 8 minutes. Flip; cook until a thermometer inserted in burger reads 160°, 6-8 minutes longer. Serve burgers on buns, with toppings as desired.

# Air-Fryer Acorn Squash Slices

**TOTAL TIME: Prep: 15 min. Cook: 15 min./batch  Servings: 6**

**INGREDIENTS**

- 2 medium acorn squash
- 2/3 cup packed brown sugar
- 1/2 cup butter, softened

**DIRECTIONS**

1. Preheat air fryer to 350°. Cut squash in half lengthwise; remove and discard seeds. Cut each half crosswise into 1/2-in. slices; discard ends. In batches, arrange squash in a single layer on greased tray in air-fryer basket. Cook until just tender, 5 minutes per side.
2. Combine sugar and butter; spread over squash. Cook 3 minutes longer.

# Air Fryer Tortellini with Prosciutto

**TOTAL TIME: Prep: 25 min. Cook: 10 min./batch Servings: 3-1/2**

## INGREDIENTS

- 1 tablespoon olive oil
- 3 tablespoons finely chopped onion
- 4 garlic cloves, coarsely chopped
- 1 can (15 ounces) tomato puree
- 1 tablespoon minced fresh basil
- 1/4 teaspoon salt
- 1/4 teaspoon pepper

**TORTELLINI:**

- 2 large eggs
- 2 tablespoons 2% milk
- 2/3 cup seasoned bread crumbs
- 1 teaspoon garlic powder
- 2 tablespoons grated pecorino Romano cheese
- 1 tablespoon minced fresh parsley
- 1/2 teaspoon salt
- 1 package (12 ounces) refrigerated prosciutto ricotta tortellini
- Cooking spray

## DIRECTIONS

1. In a small saucepan, heat oil over medium-high heat. Add onion and garlic; cook and stir until tender, 3-4 minutes. Stir in tomato puree, basil, salt and pepper. Bring to a boil; reduce heat. Simmer, uncovered, 10 minutes. Keep warm.
2. Meanwhile, preheat air fryer to 350°. In a small bowl, whisk eggs and milk. In another bowl, combine bread crumbs, garlic powder, cheese, parsley and salt.
3. Dip tortellini in egg mixture, then in bread crumb mixture to coat. In batches, arrange tortellini in a single layer on greased tray in air-fryer basket; spritz with cooking spray. Cook until golden brown, 4-5 minutes. Turn; spritz with cooking spray. Cook until golden brown, 4-5 minutes longer. Serve with sauce; sprinkle with additional minced fresh basil.

◇◇◇◇◇◇◇◇◇◇◇◇◇◇◇◇◇◇◇◇◇◇◇◇◇◇◇◇◇◇◇◇◇◇◇◇◇◇◇◇

# Air-Fryer Cumin Carrots

**TOTAL TIME: Prep: 20 min. Cook: 15 min. Servings: 4**

## INGREDIENTS

- 2 teaspoons coriander seeds
- 2 teaspoons cumin seeds
- 1 pound carrots, peeled and cut into 41/2-inch sticks
- 1 tablespoon melted coconut oil or butter
- 2 garlic cloves, minced
- 1/4 teaspoon salt
- 1/8 teaspoon pepper
- Minced fresh cilantro, optional

## DIRECTIONS

1. 1. Preheat air fryer to 325°. In a dry small skillet, toast coriander and cumin seeds over medium heat 45-60 seconds or until aromatic, stirring frequently. Cool slightly. Grind in a spice grinder, or with a mortar and pestle, until finely crushed.
2. 2. Place carrots in a large bowl. Add melted coconut oil, garlic, salt, pepper and crushed spices; toss to coat. Place on greased tray in air-fryer basket.
3. 3. Cook until crisp-tender and lightly browned, 12-15 minutes, stirring occasionally. If desired, sprinkle with cilantro.

# Air-Fryer Peppermint Lava Cakes

**TOTAL TIME: Takes: 30 min. Servings: 4**

**INGREDIENTS**

- 2/3 cup semisweet chocolate chips
- 1/2 cup butter, cubed
- 1 cup confectioners' sugar
- 2 large eggs, room temperature
- 2 large egg yolks, room temperature
- 1 teaspoon peppermint extract
- 6 tablespoons all-purpose flour
- 2 tablespoons finely crushed peppermint candies, optional

**DIRECTIONS**

1. Preheat air fryer to 375°. In a microwave-safe bowl, melt chocolate chips and butter for 30 seconds; stir until smooth. Whisk in confectioners' sugar, eggs, egg yolks and extract until blended. Fold in flour.
2. Generously grease and flour four 4-oz. ramekins; pour batter into ramekins. Do not overfill. Place ramekins on tray in air-fryer basket; cook until a thermometer reads 160° and edges of cakes are set, 10-12 minutes. Do not overcook.
3. Remove from basket; let stand 5 minutes. Carefully run a knife around sides of ramekins several times to loosen cake; invert onto dessert plates. Sprinkle with crushed candies. Serve immediately.

# Air-Fryer Brats with Beer Gravy

**TOTAL TIME: Prep/Total Time: 20 min. Servings: 5**

**INGREDIENTS**

- 1 package uncooked bratwurst links (20 ounces)
- 2 tablespoons butter
- 1 medium onion, thinly sliced
- 2 tablespoons all-purpose flour
- 1/8 teaspoon dill weed
- 1/8 teaspoon pepper
- 1 bottle (12 ounces) beer or nonalcoholic beer
- 5 slices thick bread

**DIRECTIONS**

1. Preheat air fryer to 400°. Place bratwurst in a single layer in a greased air fryer. Cook until no longer pink, 8-10 minutes.
2. Meanwhile, in a large saucepan, heat butter over medium-high heat. Add onion; cook and stir until onions start to brown and soften. Add flour, dill weed and pepper; stir until smooth. Stir in beer. Bring to a boil. Reduce heat; simmer, stirring constantly until thickened, 3-5 minutes. To serve, place 1 brat on each slice of bread; top evenly with onion mixture.

# Air-Fryer Beefy Swiss Bundles

**TOTAL TIME: Prep: 20 min. Cook: 10 min./batch  Servings: 4**

## INGREDIENTS

- 1 pound ground beef
- 1-1/2 cups sliced fresh mushrooms
- 1/2 cup chopped onion
- 1-1/2 teaspoons minced garlic
- 4 teaspoons Worcestershire sauce
- 3/4 teaspoon dried rosemary, crushed
- 3/4 teaspoon paprika
- 1/2 teaspoon salt
- 1/4 teaspoon pepper
- 1 sheet frozen puff pastry, thawed
- 2/3 cup refrigerated mashed potatoes
- 1 cup shredded Swiss cheese
- 1 large egg
- 2 tablespoons water

## DIRECTIONS

1. Preheat air fryer to 375°. In a large skillet, cook beef, mushrooms and onion over medium heat until meat is no longer pink and vegetables are tender, 8-10 minutes; crumble meat. Add garlic; cook 1 minute longer. Drain. Stir in Worcestershire sauce and seasonings. Remove from the heat; set aside.
2. On a lightly floured surface, roll puff pastry into a 15x13-in. rectangle. Cut into four 7-1/2x6-1/2-in. rectangles. Place about 2 tablespoons potatoes over each rectangle; spread to within 1 in. of edges. Top each with 3/4 cup beef mixture; sprinkle with 1/4 cup cheese.
3. Beat egg and water; brush wash over pastry edges. Bring opposite corners of pastry over each bundle; pinch seams to seal. Brush with remaining egg mixture. In batches, place pastries in a single layer on tray in air-fryer basket; cook until golden brown, 10-12 minutes.

# BEST AIR FRYER RECIPES THAT PROVE IT MAKES EVERYTHING SO MUCH TASTIER

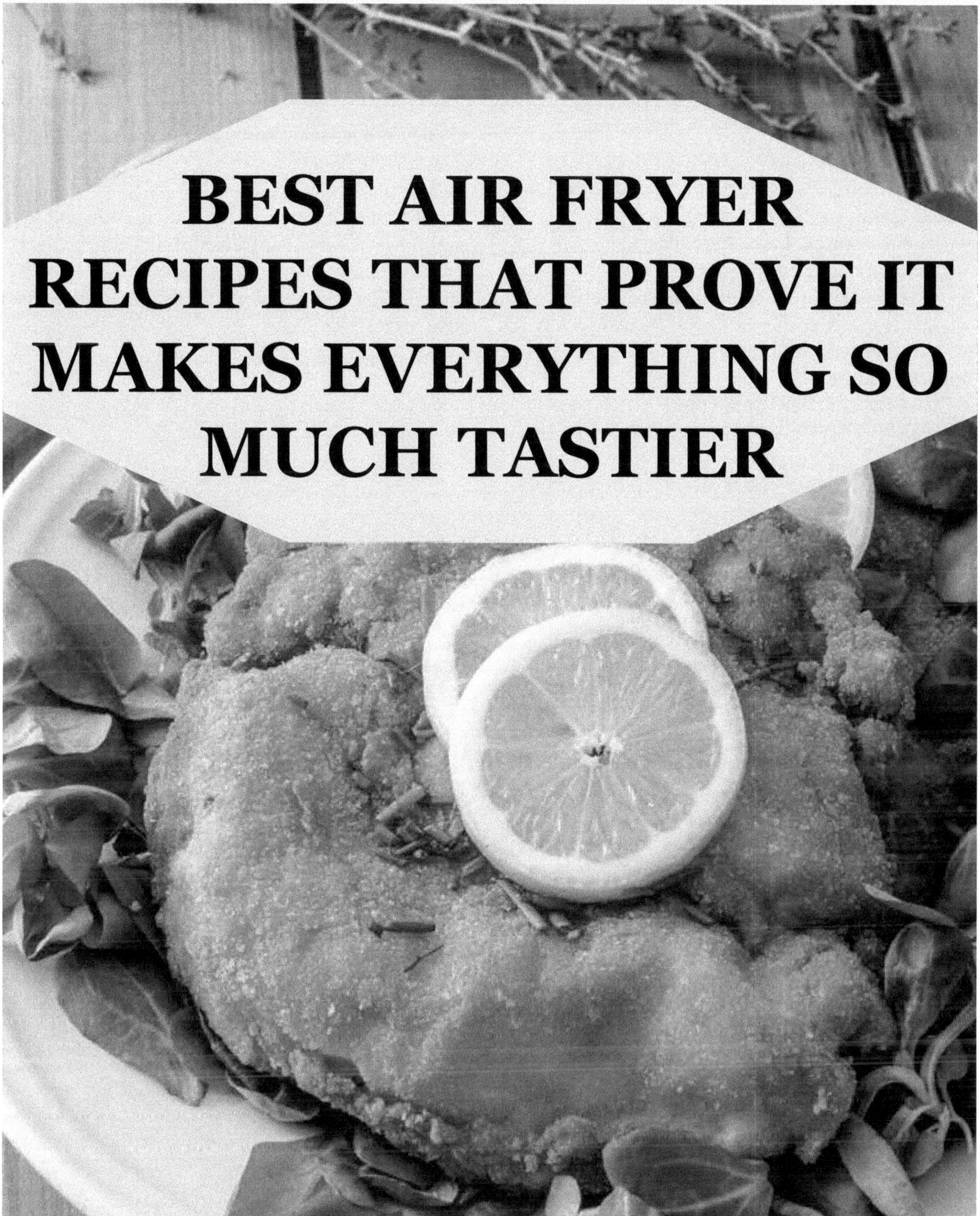

# Air Fryer Cauliflower with Cilantro Yogurt Sauce

**Prep Time: 10 minutes  Cook Time: 15 minutes  Servings: 4**

## INGREDIENTS

**For the Cauliflower**

- 1 Cauliflower (Gobi) medium, rinsed & cut into florets (about 1.25 lbs or 5 cups)
- 2 tablespoon Oil I used Avocado oil
- 1/2 teaspoon Garlic powder
- 1/2 teaspoon Ground Cumin (Jeera powder)
- 1/2 teaspoon Kosher Salt adjust to taste
- 1/4 teaspoon Black Pepper

**For the Sauce**

- 1/2 cup Fresh Cilantro chopped
- 1/4 cup Yogurt plain, greek yogurt works well too
- 1 Green chili pepper or jalapeno (seeds removed), adjust to taste
- 1 clove Garlic peeled
- 1/2 teaspoon Ground Cumin (Jeera powder)
- 1/2 teaspoon Kosher Salt
- 1/2 teaspoon Lime juice

## DIRECTIONS

**For the cauliflower**

1. In a large bowl, combine all the ingredients for the cauliflower - cauliflower florets, oil, garlic powder, cumin, coriander and salt. Toss until well combined.
2. Cauliflower mixed with spices and oil
3. Transfer the spiced cauliflower to the air fryer basket. Make sure they are spread in a single layer.
4. cauliflower mixed with oil and spices in an air fryer basket
5. Set the air fryer at 380F for 15 minutes.
6. Roasted cauliflower in the air fryer
7. For the cilantro yogurt sauce
8. While the cauliflower is cooking, add all the sauce ingredients in a small blender or food processor - cilantro, yogurt, green chili pepper, garlic, cumin, salt and lime juice.
9. Blend to a sauce. Add 1-2 tablespoons of water as needed to blend.
10. Serving
11. After the air fryer cooking time is done and the cauliflower is roasted, transfer to a serving plate. Drizzle the sauce over the cauliflower. Any leftover sauce can be used as a dip for the cauliflower. Serve right away!

# Air Fryer Lemon Garlic Salmon

**Prep Time: 5 minutes  Cook Time: 11 minutes  Servings: 4**

## INGREDIENTS

- 4 6 oz salmon filets
- 2 tbsp olive oil
- 2 tsp garlic powder
- 1 tsp celtic sea salt
- 1 tsp fresh cracked pepper
- 1 lemon, sliced into thin rounds
- 1 tsp lemon juice (I put a flexible cutting board down when slicing my lemon, as I'll usually just use the juice that comes from cutting it.)
- 2 tsp Italian herbs

## DIRECTIONS

1. In a large bowl, drizzle lemon juice and olive oil over salmon and rub to make sure the salmon filets are evenly coated.
2. Season generously with salt, pepper, and Italian herbs.
3. Arrange salmon filets in air fryer basket, making sure they dont touch too much (don"t over crowd the basket, so air can move around salmon easily).
4. Arrange lemon slices on and around salmon in air fryer basket.
5. Set air fryer to 400 degrees and cook for 10 minutes for salmon with a little bit of red in the middle.
6. Cook for 12 minutes for salmon with no red in the middle, 14 for well done salmon or thicker salmon filets.
7. Serve and enjoy!

◇◇◇◇◇◇◇◇◇◇◇◇◇◇◇◇◇◇◇◇◇◇◇◇◇◇◇◇◇◇◇◇◇◇◇◇◇◇◇◇

# Air Fryer Pasta Chips

**Prep Time: 7 minutes  Cook Time: 10 minutes  Servings: 4**

## INGREDIENTS

- 200 g short pasta (I've used Farfalle)
- 3 tbsp extra virgin olive oil
- 1 tsp dried oregano or Italian seasoning
- 1 tsp garlic powder
- 20 g Parmigiano Reggiano Cheese
- Chilli flakes (optional)

## DIRECTIONS

1. In a large pot, boil pasta in salted water as per the packet instructions. They should be cooked just over aldente
2. Drain and place into a bowl. Season with olive oil, oregano, garlic powder and chili flakes (optional)
3. Grate in the parmesan cheese and mix well so all the pasta is nicely coated

**Air Fryer Pasta Chips**

4. Cook in a preheated airfryer for 10-12 minutes at 180°C/350°F, shaking half way until they are golden brown
5. Oven Baked Pasta Chips
6. Place pasta on a baking tray lined with a baking sheet or parchment paper.
7. Spread the pasta out so that they aren't overlapping or touching.
8. Bake at 200°C/400°F for 17 - 20 minutes (depending on oven strength) until they are nice and golden brown
9. Serve with your favourite sauce, this can be either a napoletana sauce, pesto or even hummus!

# Air Fryer Southern Fried Chicken

**Prep Time**: **20 minutes** **Cook Time**: **20 minutes** **Servings**: **6**

## INGREDIENTS

- 2 lbs. chicken I used 6 legs

**Spice Mix**

- 2 teaspoons sea salt
- 1 1/2 teaspoons black pepper
- 1 1/2 teaspoons garlic powder
- 1 1/2 teaspoons paprika
- 1 teaspoon onion powder
- 1 teaspoon Italian Seasoning
- 1 cup self-rising flour
- 1/4 cup cornstarch
- 2 eggs room temperature
- 1 tablespoon hot sauce
- 2 tablespoons milk or buttermilk
- 1/4 cup water
- olive oil

## DIRECTIONS

1. Wash and dry chicken, set aside.
2. In a bowl combine seasonings.
3. Coat chicken generously with about a tablespoon of the spice mixture. (Add a splash of olive oil to the chicken to help distribute the spices if needed. Really rub it in!). Set aside.
4. In a gallon-size plastic bag, mix together flour, cornstarch, and remaining spice mix. (VERY IMPORTANT: Flour SHOULD taste well-seasoned. Add in more spices and salt if needed) Set aside.
5. In a large dish, mix together eggs, hot sauce, milk, and water.
6. Coat chicken very lightly in the flour mixture, shaking off the excess.
7. Place on a tray to allow time for some of the flour to absorb a little.
8. Coat the chicken in the egg mixture (shaking off excess).
9. Immediately, coat the chicken lightly in the flour mixture, shaking off excess.
10. Let chicken rest for about 15 minutes so that some of the flour is absorbed.
11. Use an oil mister or brush, to coat the chicken very lightly (all over) with olive oil.
12. Place chicken in greased Air Fryer basket, allowing room for the air to flow all around the chicken. (do not crowd)
13. Cook according to your air fryer, flipping halfway and brushing very lightly with more oil (if needed) so that no flour is visible. (I cooked on 350 F. for about 18 minutes)
14. Remove and let chicken rest for about 5 minutes.
15. Serve immediately. (Homemade air fried chicken does not stay crisp very long)

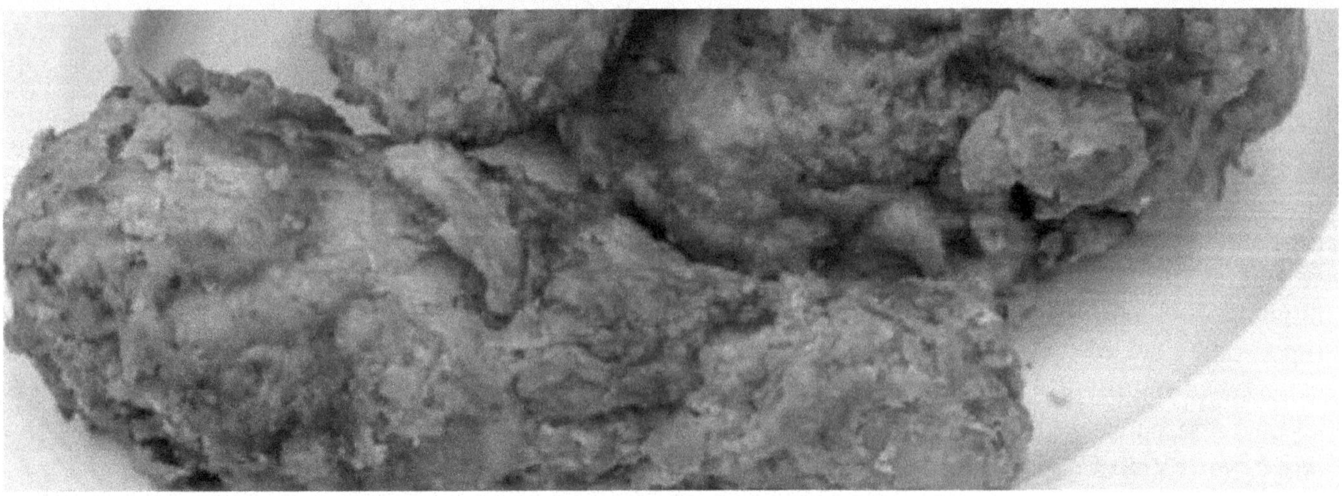

## Air Fryer Everything Bagels

**Prep Time**: **10 minutes** **Cook Time**: **30 minutes** **Servings**: **4**

### INGREDIENTS

- 1 cup unbleached all-purpose flour plus more for dusting work surface
- 2¼ teaspoon baking powder
- 1/2 teaspoon kosher salt
- 1/2 teaspoon onion powder
- 1/4 teaspoon garlic powder
- 2 tablespoons sunflower seeds unsalted shelled
- 1 cup plain nonfat greek yogurt
- 1 egg beaten
- 1 splash water

[homemade everything seasoning]

### DIRECTIONS

1. In a bowl, measure and add the flour, baking powder, salt, onion and garlic powder. Whisk to combine.
2. Add in the sunflower seeds and stir.
3. Next, add in the greek yogurt, switch over to a rubber spatula and mix until combined. Shape into a ball and turn out onto a floured surface.
4. Divide the dough into 4 equal parts. Roll each piece in a little flour before rolling into a 10-inch rope.
5. Place a sheet of parchment onto a plate or rimmed baking sheet. Sprinkle a little of the everything seasoning over top.
6. Place each bagel onto the seasoning and gently press. Reshaping the bagel if necessary.
7. Thoroughly beat the egg with a splash of water. Brush the tops and sides of the bagel with the egg wash before sprinkling with more everything seasoning.
8. Preheat your air fryer to 300°. Depending on the size, you may need to work in batches. Air fry bagels for 12 to 15 minutes.
9. Allow to cool sligthly before slicing and toasting.

◇◇◇◇◇◇◇◇◇◇◇◇◇◇◇◇◇◇◇◇◇◇◇◇◇◇◇◇◇◇◇◇◇◇◇◇◇◇◇

## Air Fryer Jerk Pork

**Prep Time: 10 minutes** **Cook Time: 20 minutes** **Servings: 4**

### INGREDIENTS

- 1.5 lbs pork butt chopped into large 3 inch pieces
- ¼ cup jerk paste
- oil for spraying basket

### DIRECTIONS

1. Rub pork pieces with jerk paste and allow it to marinate pork for 4-24 hours in the refrigerator. The longer the better.
2. Preheat air fryer to 390 degrees F. Spray the bottom of the basket to ensure they dont stick.
3. Remove pork and allow to rest at room temp for 20 minutes. Place in air fryer ensuring they are spaced apart. Set time for 20 minutes, flip halfway.
4. Remove from air fryer and allow to sit for 5-10 minutes before cutting.
5. Enjoy.

# Air Fryer Hush Puppies

**Prep Time**: **10 minutes** **Cook Time**: **9 minutes** **Servings**: **18 - 20**

## INGREDIENTS

- 1 cup (130 grams) all-purpose flour
- 1 cup (120 grams) cornmeal
- ½ tablespoon (6 grams) baking powder
- 2 tablespoons (25 grams) sugar
- 1 teaspoon (8grams) salt
- 1 tablespoon garlic powder
- 1/3 cup (80 grams) buttermilk
- 1 large egg
- 2-3 tablespoons chopped or grated onion
- 2-3 tablespoons chopped green onions
- 3 tablespoons (40 grams) unsalted butter

## DIRECTIONS

1. In a medium bowl, whisk together the flour, cornmeal, baking powder, sugar, salt, and garlic powder
2. In another bowl, whisk in buttermilk, and lightly beaten eggs until well combined.
3. Add the dry ingredients with the wet ingredients until fully incorporated, then add grated onions and butter.
4. Preheat the Air Fryer - I preheat mine at 400 Degrees/ 204 degrees C for 5 minutes when ready to air fry.
5. Lightly grease the metal basket with cooking spray and arrange hush puppies in a single layer without touching each other.
6. Set your Air Fryer to 380°F, for 4-5 minutes. Flip over carefully and cook on the other side for an additional 4 minutes, or until cooked through and hush puppy is crispy.
7. Serve with this fried fish or remoulade sauce.

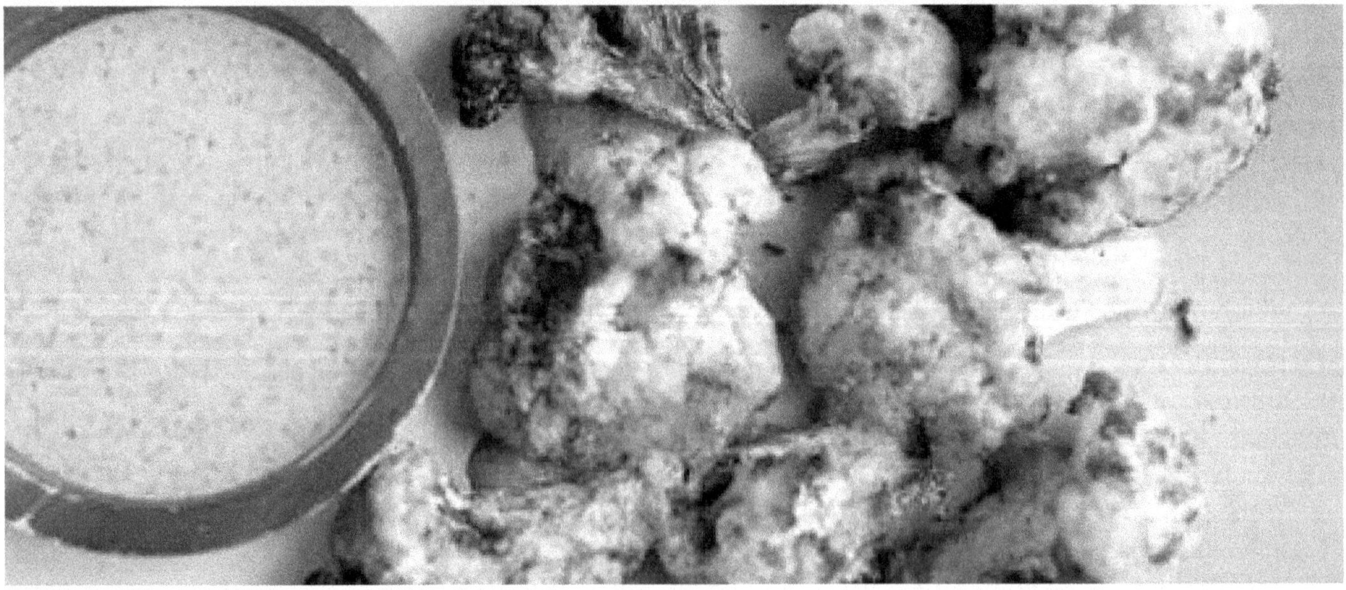

# Air Fryer Buffalo Chicken Wings

**Servings: 4**

## INGREDIENTS

- 12 pieces 26 ounces chicken wing portions (a mix of drumettes and wingettes)
- 6 tablespoons Frank's RedHot sauce
- 2 tablespoons distilled white vinegar
- 1 teaspoon dried oregano
- 1 teaspoon garlic powder
- 1/2 teaspoon kosher salt

**Blue Cheese Dip**

- 1/4 cup crumbled blue cheese
- 1/3 cup 2% Greek yogurt
- 1/2 tablespoon fresh lemon juice
- 1/2 tablespoon distilled white vinegar
- For Serving
- 2 celery stalks, halved crosswise and cut into 8 sticks total
- 2 medium carrots, peeled, halved crosswise and cut into 8 sticks total

## DIRECTIONS

1. In a large bowl, combine the chicken with 1 tablespoon of the hot sauce, the vinegar, oregano, garlic powder, and salt, tossing to coat well.
2. For the blue cheese dip: In a small bowl, mash the blue cheese and yogurt together with a fork. Stir in the lemon juice and vinegar until well blended. Refrigerate until ready to serve.
3. Preheat the air fryer to 400°F.
4. Working in batches, arrange a single layer of the chicken in the air fryer basket. Cook for 22 minutes, flipping halfway, until crispy, browned, and cooked through. (For a toaster oven-style air fryer, the temperature remains the same; cook for 15 16 minutes.) Transfer to a large clean bowl (do not use the bowl the marinade was in.) When all the batches are done, return all the chicken to the air fryer and cook for 1 minute to heat through.
5. Return the chicken to the bowl and toss with the remaining 5 tablespoons hot sauce to coat. Arrange on a platter and serve with the celery, carrot sticks, and blue cheese dip.

# Air Fryer Reuben Stromboli

**Prep Time: 10 minutes  Cook Time: 15 minutes  Servings: 6**

## INGREDIENTS

- 12 ounces fresh pizza dough
- 1 tablespoon Thousand Island dressing
- 1/2 pound thinly sliced corned beef
- 6 slices swiss cheese
- 1 cup sauerkraut, squeezed in paper towels to get rid of liquid
- Thousand Island for serving
- cooking spray
- 1/4 teaspoon garlic salt

## DIRECTIONS

1. Roll dough into a rectangles about 10 inches long. Spread Thousand Island over the top.
2. Layer the corned beef, sauerkraut, and cheese, leaving a 1-inch border.
3. Starting on one long side, roll the dough up. Stretch the ends and tuck them under. Position so seam is on bottom. Lightly spray top with cooking spray and sprinkle with garlic salt.
4. Set Air Fryer to 350 for 15 minutes. Let preheat for 2 minutes. Place stromboli in the Air Fryer basket and Air Fry for the remaning 13 minutes.
5. Cut into slices and serve with Thousand Island dressing.

◇◇◇◇◇◇◇◇◇◇◇◇◇◇◇◇◇◇◇◇◇◇◇◇◇◇◇◇◇◇◇◇◇◇◇◇◇◇◇◇

# Air Fryer Fried Green Tomatoes

**Prep Time: 5 minutes  Cook Time: 8 minutes  Servings: 4**

## INGREDIENTS

- 2 green tomatoes, (3 if they are smaller)
- salt and pepper
- 1/2 cup all-purpose flour
- 2 large eggs
- 1/2 cup buttermilk
- 1 cup Panko crumbs
- 1 cup yellow cornmeal
- n=mister filled with olive oil or vegetable oil

## DIRECTIONS

1. Cut tomatoes into 1/4-inch slices. Pat dry with paper towels and season well with salt and pepper.
2. Place flour in a shallow dish or pie plate, or for easy clean-up use a paper plate.
3. Whisk together eggs and buttermilk in a shallow dish or bowl.
4. Combine Panko crumbs and cornmeal in a shallow dish or pie plate, or for easy clean-up use a paper plate.
5. Preheat air fryer to 400 degrees.
6. Coat the tomato slices in the flour, dip in egg mixture, and then press panko crumb mixture into both sides. Sprinkle a little more salt on them.
7. Mist air fryer basket with oil and place 4 tomato slices in basket. Mist the tops with oil. Air-fry for 5 minutes.
8. Flip tomatoes over, mist with oil and air-fry 3 more minutes.
9. Serve with Comeback sauce if desired.

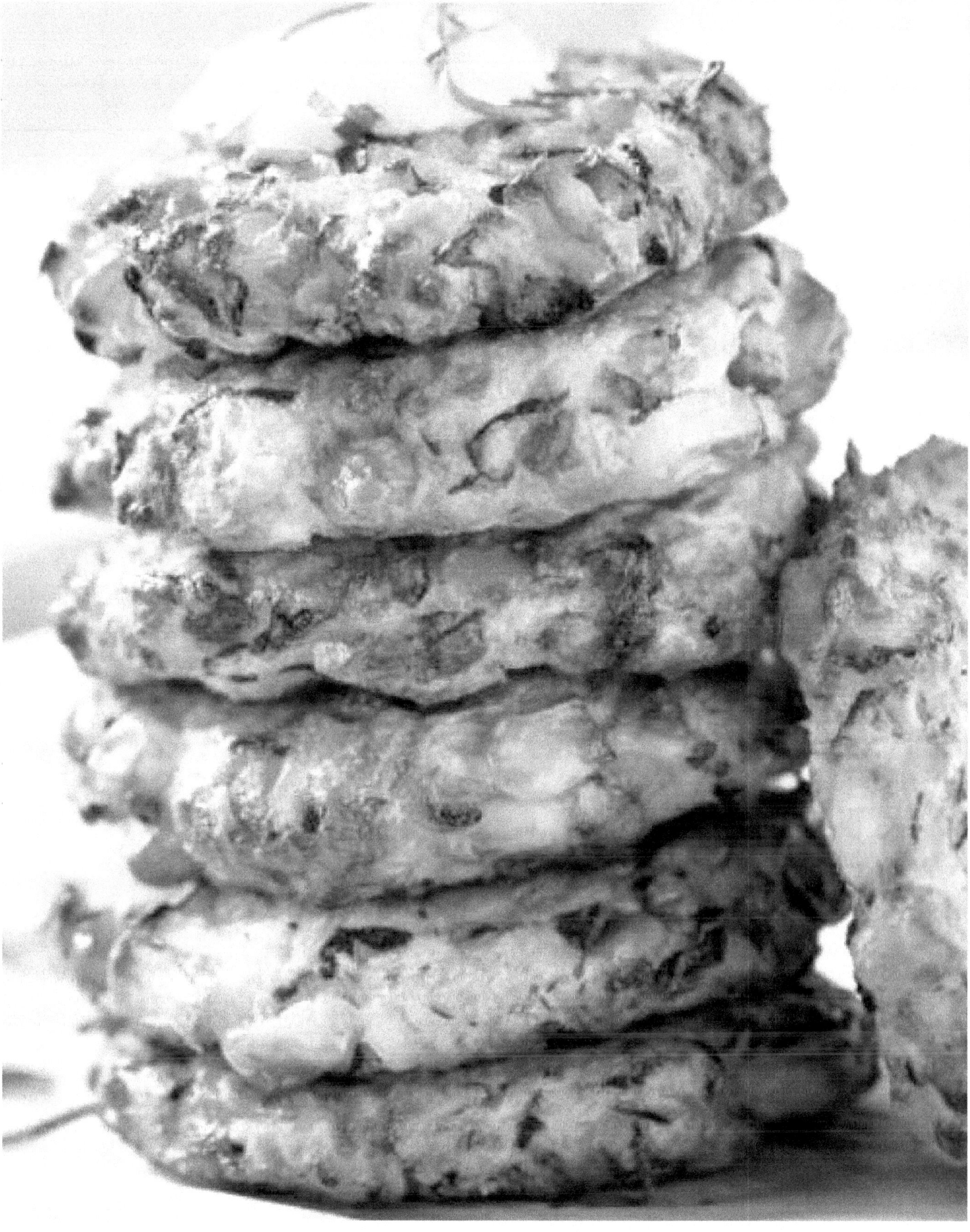

# Air Fryer Meatloaf

**Prep Time**: **15 minutes** **Cook Time**: **35 minutes** **Resting Time**: **10 minutes**
**Servings**: **6**

## INGREDIENTS

- 1 lb Protein I used Beyond Meat, you can use beef, turkey, pork, etc
- 1/2 c breadcrumbs (or ½ c flour) *if you are gluten free, use gf
- 2 T ketchup
- 1/2 cup onion diced
- 1/4 c fresh parsley
- 1 egg whisked
- 1 T mustard
- 1 T liquid smoke
- 1 t garlic powder
- 1/2 t salt
- 1/2 t smoked paprika
- 1/2 t oregano
- Glaze
- 1/4 c ketchup
- 1/4 c brown sugar
- 2 t Dijon mustard

## DIRECTIONS

1. To make your air fryer meatloaf, start with your protein in a bowl. The process is basically a dump and stir. The items can be added in any order.
2. Add the breadcrumbs. Fold in the onions. Add the spices.
3. Pour in the fresh diced parsley. Add the scrambled egg. Pour in the ketchup, mustard and liquid smoke. Stir well to combine.
4. Shape mixture into a loaf shape. Put air fryer meatloaf into the air fryer basket on top of parchment paper.
5. Air Fry for 20 minutes at 370 degrees F.
6. Remove the air fryer basket from the unit. Mix the glaze ingredients together. Spread the glaze on top of the air fryer meatloaf.
7. Return meatloaf back to the air fryer unit and continue cooking at the same temperature for 10-15 minutes. (If you are using meat, it needs to reach 165 degrees F minimum, use your meat thermometer).
8. Let air fryer meatloaf stand still for 10 minutes. This will help the ingredients to unify and it will help when you go to cut it.
9. ENJOY!

# Air Fryer Egg Rolls

**Prep Time: 5 minutes  Cook Time: 50 minutes  Servings: 4 - 6**

## INGREDIENTS

- 1 tbsp. sesame oil
- 1/2 lb. ground pork
- 4 c. coleslaw mix
- 1/2 c. matchstick-cut carrots
- 1 tsp. freshly grated ginger
- 2 garlic cloves, minced
- 3 green onions, sliced
- 2 tsp. soy sauce
- 2 tsp. rice vinegar
- 1/2 tsp. ground black pepper
- 1/4 tsp. kosher salt
- 1/8 tsp. Chinese 5-spice seasoning
- 12 egg roll wrappers
- Nonstick cooking spray
- 1 tbsp. olive oil
- Sweet chili sauce, duck sauce, or hot mustard sauce, for dipping

## DIRECTIONS

1. Heat the sesame oil in a large skillet over medium heat. Add the pork and cook until crumbled and cooked through, about 4 minutes. Add the coleslaw mix, carrots, ginger and garlic. Cook 2-3 minutes or until the cabbage has wilted. Remove from the heat; stir in the green onions, soy sauce, vinegar, pepper, salt, and 5-spice seasoning. Transfer to a plate and let cool slightly.
2. Place 1 egg roll wrapper on a dry work surface with the points of the wrapper facing up and down (like a diamond). Place about 1/3 cup of the pork mixture in the middle of the wrapper. Dip your fingers in water and and dampen the edges of the wrapper. Fold the left then right points of the wrapper in toward the center. Fold the bottom point over the center. Roll toward the remaining point to form a tight cylinder. Press edges to seal. Place on a plate and cover with a dry towel. Repeat the process with remaining wrappers and pork mixture.
3. Preheat the air fryer to 360°, if required. Spray the air fryer basket with cooking spray. Brush the tops of the egg rolls with olive oil. Working in 3 batches (4 at a time), place the egg rolls in the basket and cook 7 minutes. Flip the egg rolls over and brush with more oil. Cook for an additional 2 minutes.
4. Serve with the dipping sauce of your choice.

# Air Fryer Roast Beef

**Prep Time: 5 minutes    Cook Time: 35 minutes    Servings: 7**

## INGREDIENTS

- 2 lb beef roast top round or eye of round is best
- oil for spraying
- Rub
- 1 tbs kosher salt
- 1 tsp black pepper
- 2 tsp garlic powder
- 1 tsp summer savory OR thyme

## DIRECTIONS

1. Mix all rub ingredients and rub into roast.
2. Place fat side down in the basket of the air fryer (or set up for rotisserie if your air fryer is so equipped)
3. Lightly spray with oil.
4. Set fryer to 400 degrees F and air fry for 20 minutes; turn fat-side up and spray lightly with oil. Continue cooking for 15 additional minutes at 400 degrees F.
5. Remove the roast from the fryer, tent with foil and let the meat rest for 10 minutes.
6. The time given should produce a rare roast which should be 125 degrees F on a meat thermometer. Additional time will be needed for medium, medium-well and well. Always use a meat thermometer to test the temperature.
7. Approximate times for medium and well respectively are 40 minutes and 45 minutes. Remember to always use a meat thermometer as times are approximate and fryers differ by wattage.

◇◇◇◇◇◇◇◇◇◇◇◇◇◇◇◇◇◇◇◇◇◇◇◇◇◇◇◇◇◇◇◇◇◇◇◇◇◇◇◇

# Air Fryer Pizza

**Prep Time: 10 minutes    Cook Time: 10 minutes    Servings: 2**

## INGREDIENTS

- 1 pkg pizza dough mix 6.5 oz. , used Betty Crocker mix with water
- 1/4 c spaghetti sauce
- 1/2-3/4 c mozzarella cheese
- pepperoni optional
- olives optional
- olive oil spray

## DIRECTIONS

1. Preheat your air fryer at 320 degrees for 3 minutes.
2. Make your pizza dough. Spray 7" springform pan and spread dough inside so it is level across the pan.
3. Put into air fryer and spray top of raw pizza dough with olive oil.
4. Close lid/drawer and set to 320 degrees for 3 minutes so dough can cook a bit.
5. Open and add pizza sauce, cheese, pepperoni and other toppings.
6. Close lid/drawer again and reset to 320 degrees for 7 minutes. Add 1 more minute if you want top crispier. Enjoy!

# Air Fryer Sour Cream and Onion Chicken

**Prep Time**: **10 minutes** **Cook Time**: **10 minutes** **Servings**: **4**

## INGREDIENTS

Marinade

- 4 skinless boneless chicken breasts halved to make 4 breasts
- 1/4 cup fresh parsley chopped
- 1/2 cup sour cream plus an additional 2 tablespoons
- 2 tsp onion powder
- 1 1/2 tbsp chives
- 1 1/2 tbsp green onions
- 1/2 tbsp fresh lemon juice
- 2 1/2 tsp salt and pepper
- 1 tsp sugar
- cooking spray
- For the dredge
- 1 3/4 cups Panko breadcrumbs
- 1/4 cup parmesan
- 1 tsp lemon zest
- 1 egg

## DIRECTIONS

1. Add all of the marinade ingredients to a plastic zip bag or bowl. Mix well. Add the chicken. Make sure to coat the chicken all over with the marinade. Zip the bag up. Place it into the fridge and marinate overnight.
2. Let the chicken come to room temperature.
3. Add the egg to a shallow bowl. Lightly beat it. In a separate shallow bowl add the bread crumbs, Parmesan cheese and lemon zest. Mix to combine.
4. Dip both sides of the chicken into the eggs. Let excess drip back into the bowl. Next, dip the chicken into the panko crumbs. Cover both sides with panko, pressing very well to adhere. Shake off excess. *See notes below.
5. Spray some oil into the air fryer. Place chicken in the air fryer. Spray the top of chicken with a bit of the oil.
6. Set air fryer to 400 @ 5 minutes per side or until internal temperature reaches 165 degrees Fahrenheit. Cooking times will vary depending on the thickness and size of breast.

◇◇◇◇◇◇◇◇◇◇◇◇◇◇◇◇◇◇◇◇◇◇◇◇◇◇◇◇◇◇◇◇◇◇◇◇◇◇◇◇◇

# Air Fryer Fried Pickles

**Prep Time**: **5 minutes** **Cook Time**: **10 minutes** **Servings: 4**

## INGREDIENTS

- 2 cups dill pickle slices
- 1/2 cup flour
- 1 large egg
- 1 Tablespoon water
- 1/2 cup bread crumbs
- 1/4 cup grated Parmesan
- 1 Tablespoon Italian seasoning

## DIRECTIONS

1. Lay the pickles on a paper towel and pat dry. In the first small bowl add the flour. In the second small bowl add the egg and whisk with the water. In the last bowl add the bread crumbs, parmesan, and italian seasoning.
2. Dip each pickle in the flour, then the egg and lastly in the bread crumb mixture.
3. Lay the pickles in a single layer in the air fryer basket. Cook at 400 degrees for 8-10 minutes. Serve with your favorite dipping sauce.

# Air Fryer Fried Chicken

**Prep Time: 15 minutes  Cook Time: 1 hr  Servings: 4**

## INGREDIENTS

- 2 pounds chicken wings chicken legs, thighs or chicken breast
- 2 cups buttermilk
- 2 large eggs
- 1 teaspoon paprika
- 1 teaspoon hot sauce
- 1 teaspoon salt or to taste
- 1 teaspoon pepper or to taste
- 2 teaspoon baking powder
- 1 ½ teaspoon baking soda
- 1 cup all-purpose flour

## DIRECTIONS

1. Prep the Chicken - Wash the chicken and pat it dry with paper towels.
2. Prepare the Buttermilk Mixture - To a large bowl add the buttermilk, eggs, paprika, hot sauce, salt, pepper and whisk until combined. Whisk in the baking powder and baking soda. In a shallow dish add the flour.
3. Dredge the Chicken - First dredge the chicken in flour on all sides, then dip into the buttermilk mixture. Dredge the chicken in flour one more time, then place the chicken on a plate or rack, and repeat with all chicken pieces.
4. Cook the Chicken - Place the chicken in the air fryer basket, allowing enough room between each piece to flow around. Spray the chicken with a bit of cooking spray or brush with oil. Cook on 375 F for about 20 minutes, flip over, spray with more cooking oil or brush with oil, and cook for another 10 minutes. Repeat with remaining chicken if doing in batches. Cooking time may vary depending on your air fryer.

◇◇◇◇◇◇◇◇◇◇◇◇◇◇◇◇◇◇◇◇◇◇◇◇◇◇◇◇◇◇◇◇◇◇◇◇◇◇◇

# Air Fryer Salsa Chicken Taquitos

**Prep Time: 5 minutes  Cook Time: 20 minutes  Servings: 20**

## INGREDIENTS

- 1 cooked chicken shredded from roasted or rotisserie chicken
- 1/2 cup salsa or more to taste
- 20 flour tortillas fajita size
- 1½ cups cheddar jack cheese
- olive oil spray

## DIRECTIONS

1. In a mixing bowl, add the shredded chicken (about 4 cups) and 1/2 to 2/3 cup of salsa or more and toss until evenly coated. Add more salsa as needed. I always eyeball it.
2. Working in batches, place a few tortillas down onto a clean surface. On 1/3 of the tortilla, place some of the salsa chicken and a little cheese.
3. Starting on the end with the chicken and cheese, fold it over and roll tightly before placing each one onto a rimmed metal baking sheet. Repeat with the remaining tortillas, chicken and cheese until all 20 are rolled.
4. Then spray all of the rolled taquitos with olive oil spray.
5. Preheat you air-fryer to 350-360° and working in batches of 4 or 5 taquitos at a time (any extra room in the basket could cause them to unroll) air-fry for 4 to 5 mintues or until crispy and golden brown.
6. Repeat with the remaining taquitos.
7. Serve as is or with desired toppings (see notes).

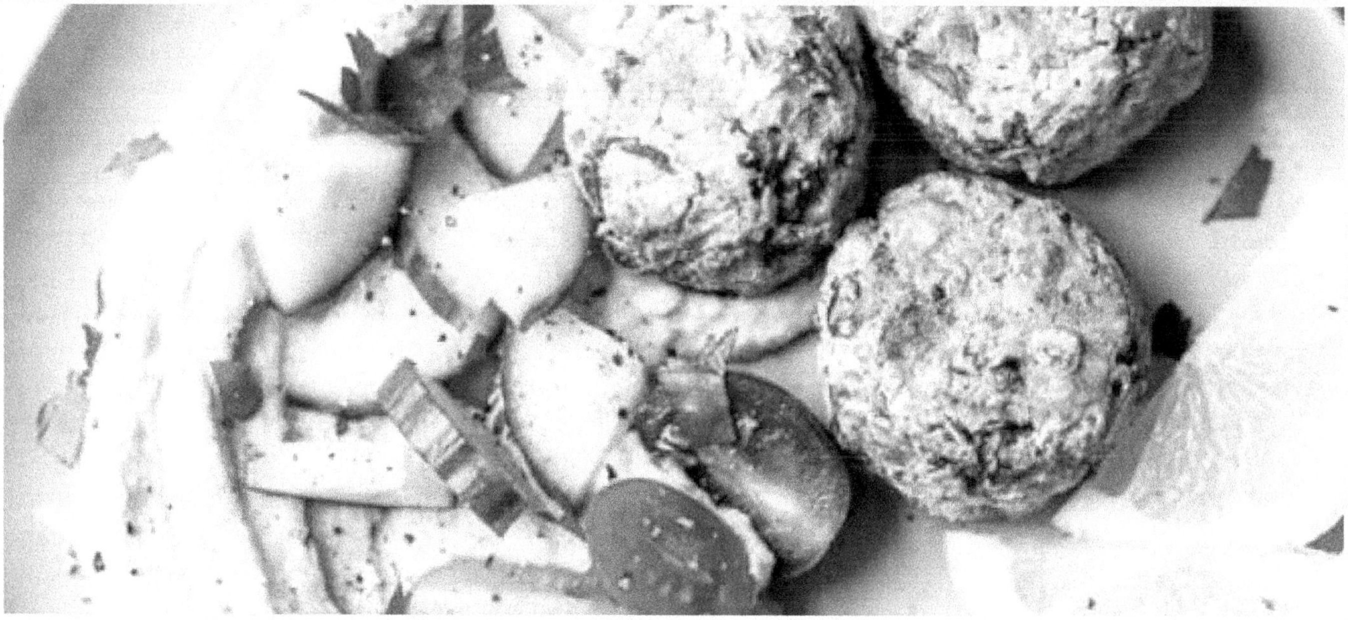

# Air Fryer Falafel

**Prep Time: 15 minutes Cook Time: 30 minutes REFRIGERATE TIME: 2 hrs**
**Servings: 4**

## INGREDIENTS

- 1 (15.5 ounce can) chickpeas, rinsed and drained
- 1 small yellow onion, quartered
- 3 cloves garlic, roughly chopped
- 1/3 cup roughly chopped parsley
- 1/3 cup roughly chopped cilantro
- 1/3 cup chopped scallions
- 1 teaspoon cumin
- 1/2 teaspoon kosher salt
- 1/8 teaspoon crushed red pepper flakes
- 1 teaspoon baking powder
- 4 tablespoons all purpose flour, plus more for dusting
- olive oil spray

**Optional for serving:**

- hummus, sliced tomatoes, sliced cucumber, thinly sliced red onion, pita, tahini, etc

## DIRECTIONS

1. Dry the chickpeas on paper towels.
2. Place the onions and garlic in the bowl of a food processor fitted with a steel blade. Add the parsley, scallions, cilantro, cumin, salt, and red pepper flakes.
3. Process until blended 30 to 60 seconds, then add the chickpeas and pulse 2 to 3 times until just blended, but not pureed.
4. Sprinkle in the baking powder and the flour, scrape the sides of the bowl down with a spatula and pulse 2 to 3 times.
5. Transfer to a bowl and refrigerate, covered, 2 to 3 hours.
6. Form the falafel mixture into 12 balls, if it's too sticky add some flour to your hands and your work surface.
7. Preheat the air fryer 350F.
8. Spray the falafel with oil. Cook 14 minutes, in batches until golden brown, turning halfway.

# Air Fryer Chicken Cordon Bleu

**Prep Time: 10 minutes** **Cook Time: 30 minutes** **Servings: 6**

## INGREDIENTS

### Chicken

- 3 chicken breasts filled to form 6 thin pieces of chicken
- 6 slices ham turkey ham also works great
- 6 slices swiss cheese
- 1/2 cup bread crumbs
- 1/2 cup panko bread crumbs
- toothpicks
- cooking spray

### Sauce

- 2 tbsp butter
- 2 tbsp flour
- 3/4 cup milk
- 3/4 cup chicken broth
- 1/2 tsp salt
- pepper to taste
- 1 tsp dijon mustard
- 2 tbsp grated parmesan cheese

## DIRECTIONS

1. Preheat the oven to 350. Spray a 9 x 9 baking dish with cooking spray. Mix the bread crumbs together on a plate or flat dish. To make each chicken roll up, layer one slice of ham and one slice of swiss cheese on each of the chicken pieces. Roll up tightly, then roll in the bread crumb mixture. Secure with toothpicks (I used two per piece) and place in the prepared baking dish. Spray with cooking spray. Bake 30 - 35 minutes, or until cooked through.

2. When the chicken has about 15 minutes left, make the sauce. Melt the butter in a saucepan over medium heat. Add the flour and whisk to form a smooth paste. Cook 2-3 minutes, until golden. Add the milk, whisking constantly, until combined. Cook until slightly thickened, then slowly add the chicken broth while continuing to whisk constantly to prevent lumps. Whisk in the salt and pepper. When the sauce has thickened, remove from heat and whisk in the dijon mustard and parmesan cheese until melted and combined. Serve chicken over pasta or rice and drizzle with sauce.

# Air Fryer Potatoes

**Prep Time: 5 minutes** **Cook Time: 20 minutes** **Servings: 3 - 4**

## INGREDIENTS

- 1 1/4 lb. russet potatoes, scrubbed, dried and cut into 1" pieces
- 1 tbsp. olive oil
- 1 1/2 tsp. seasoned salt
- 3/4 tsp. paprika
- 3/4 tsp. dried Italian seasoning

## DIRECTIONS

1. In a large bowl, combine the potatoes, olive oil, seasoned salt, paprika and Italian seasoning. Toss well to combine.
2. Heat an air fryer to 400 degrees for 2 minutes. Place the potatoes in the basket and cook for 10 minutes. Removing the basket and shake the potatoes. Return the potatoes to the air fryer for 8-10 more minutes, until crispy on the outside and tender on the inside. Serve immediately.

◇◇◇◇◇◇◇◇◇◇◇◇◇◇◇◇◇◇◇◇◇◇◇◇◇◇◇◇◇◇◇◇◇◇◇◇◇◇◇◇

# Air Fryer Pork Chops

**Prep Time: 10 minutes** **Cook Time: 40 minutes** **Servings: 4**

## INGREDIENTS

- 1/2 c. all-purpose flour
- 2 tsp. seasoned salt, such as Lawry's, divided
- 1/2 tsp. ground black pepper
- 1/4 tsp. cayenne pepper, optional
- 1 egg
- 1/2 c. milk
- 1 c. panko breadcrumbs
- 1/4 c. grated parmesan cheese
- 4 boneless pork loin chops (about 1" thick)
- Nonstick cooking spray
- Salad and mashed potatoes, for serving

## DIRECTIONS

1. Remove the pork chops from the refrigerator about 30 minutes before cooking. Sprinkle the chops all over with 1 teaspoon of seasoned salt, then let them come to room temperature.
2. In a shallow bowl, whisk to combine the flour, remaining 1 teaspoon of seasoned salt, black pepper and cayenne pepper. In a second shallow bowl, whisk to combine the egg and milk. In a third shallow bowl or plate, mix together the panko breadcrumbs and parmesan cheese.
3. Pat the pork chops dry with a paper towel. Dredge each of the pork chops into the flour mixture, then pat to remove any excess. Next, dip each in the egg mixture, letting any excess drip off. Finally, dredge each in the panko breadcrumb mixture and place on a clean plate. Spray both sides of the pork chops lightly with non-stick cooking spray.
4. Preheat the air fryer to 400 degrees. Place chops in a single layer in the air fryer basket and cook for 8 minutes. Flip the chops and cook for 4 more minutes, or until the internal temperature is at least 145 degrees.
5. Serve alongside a green salad and mashed potatoes.

# Air Fryer Popcorn Chicken

**Prep Time: 15 minutes** **Cook Time: 20 minutes** **Servings**: 4

## INGREDIENTS

- 2 boneless skinless chicken breasts cubed
- 2 tbsp flour
- 1 tsp garlic salt
- 1 cup buttermilk
- 1 cup panko crumbs
- pepper
- vegetable oil

## DIRECTIONS

1. Add 1-2 inches of vegetable oil to a medium pan and heat on the medium setting.
2. Mix together flour and garlic salt in a small bowl. In another small bowl add buttermilk. In a third small bowl add the panko crumbs. Place the three bowls in a line.
3. Dip the chicken pieces in the flour mixture first followed by the buttermilk and lastly the panko crumbs. Dip all the chicken pieces making sure that all sides are coated with each ingredient. NOTE: for a double coating dip the pieces in the buttermilk a second time and again in the panko crumbs. If you're make a double coating you will need extra milk and panko crumbs.
4. Place a paper towel on a plate next to the stove near the hot oil.
5. Working in batches, place the chicken pieces in the hot oil. Fry for 3-4 minutes on each side or until golden brown. Once the pieces are done use tongs to remove them from the oil and place them on the paper towel lined plate
6. Serve warm with your favorite dipping sauce.

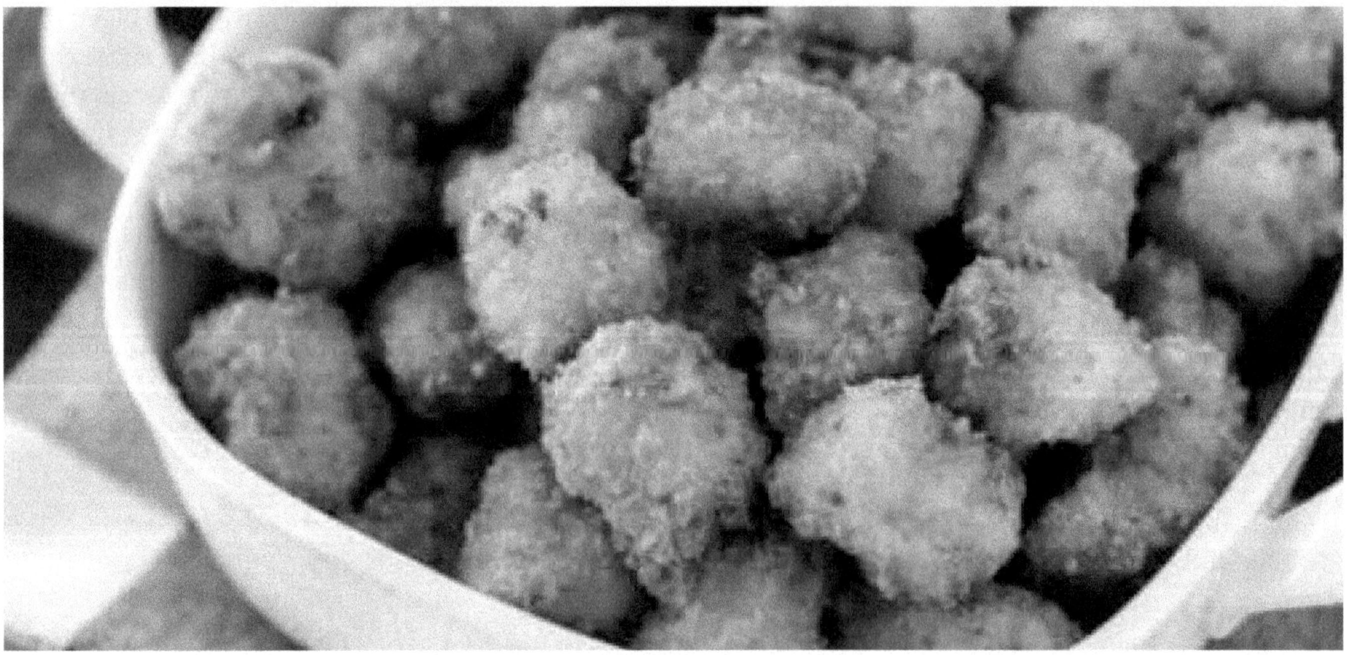

# Air Fryer Steak

**Prep Time: 5 minutes Cook Time: 40 minutes Servings: 4 - 6**

## INGREDIENTS

AIR FRYER STEAK:

- 2 lb. NY strip steaks (2 steaks, about 1 to 1 1/2-inches thick)
- 1 tbsp. olive oil
- 2 tsp. Tex-Mex seasoning blend
- 1 tsp. brown sugar
- 1/4 tsp. salt
- 1/4 tsp. ground black pepper

GARLIC-CILANTRO BUTTER:

- 3 tbsp. salted butter, softened
- 1 tbsp. fresh cilantro leaves, chopped
- 1 clove garlic, finely grated or chopped
- 1/2 tsp. lime zest
- 1/4 tsp. kosher salt
- 1/4 tsp. black pepper
- Pinch of cayenne pepper, optional

## DIRECTIONS

1. For the steaks: Remove the steaks from the refrigerator and let rest at room temperature for 30 minutes.
2. For the garlic-cilantro butter: In a small bowl, combine the softened butter, cilantro, garlic, lime zest, salt, pepper and cayenne pepper, if using. Mash with a fork to combine and mix well. Transfer the butter to a piece of plastic wrap and roll into a little log. Refrigerate for 30 minutes.
3. Meanwhile, in a small bowl, combine the Tex-Mex seasoning, brown sugar, salt and ground black pepper.
4. Brush the steaks all over with the olive oil, then sprinkle on both sides with the spice mixture.
5. Place in a single layer in an air fryer basket and cook at 400 degrees for 7 minutes. Flip the steaks and cook for an additional 3-7 minutes, or until the temperature of the steak is at around 135 degrees, for medium-rare.
6. Cut slices from the butter and set over top of the hot steak. Let rest for 5 minutes, then slice and serve.

◇◇◇◇◇◇◇◇◇◇◇◇◇◇◇◇◇◇◇◇◇◇◇◇◇◇◇◇◇◇◇◇◇◇◇◇◇◇◇◇◇

# Air Fryer Baked Sweet Potatoes

**Prep Time: 5 minutes Cook Time: 40 minutes Servings: 4**

## INGREDIENTS

- 4 medium-sized sweet potatoes scrubbed, rinsed and dried with paper towels
- 3-4 tsp olive oil
- 1 tsp kosher salt
- 1/2 tsp black pepper (optional)

## DIRECTIONS

1. Pierce sweet potatoes several times with a small knife or tines of a fork.
2. Drizzle olive oil over clean sweet potatoes and rub into potatoes with your hands to coat.
3. Sprinkle with salt and pepper (if using). Place sweet potatoes on air fryer rack or basket, making sure to leave some space between them and not stacking them
4. Cook at 390 degrees for 40-50 minutes (depending on the size of your sweet potatoes), flipping over halfway through the cook time.

# Air Fryer Stuffed Turkey Breast

**Prep Time**: **15 minutes** **Cook Time**: **45 minutes** **Servings: 8**

## INGREDIENTS

- 2 -1.5 lb. (680g) deboned turkey breasts
- salt , to taste
- black pepper , to taste

**Filling:**

- 4 slices bacon , cut into bite sized pieces
- 4 oz. (113 g) mushrooms , sliced
- 1/2 small onion , diced
- 2 cloves garlic , minced
- 2 cups (480 ml) chopped fresh kale or spinach (if frozen use 1 cup, thawed, then squeeze out water)
- 1/2 teaspoon (2.5 ml) dried thyme , oregano or rosemary (or 1/2 Tablespoon fresh)
- 1/4 teaspoon (1.25 ml) dried sage or 1/2 tablespoon fresh chopped
- 1/4 teaspoon (1.25 ml) kosher salt , or to taste
- 1/4 teaspoon (1.25 ml) black pepper , or to taste
- 1/4 cup (25 g) shredded parmesan cheese or crumbled feta
- optional - Instant Read Thermometer

## DIRECTIONS

**Make the Filling:**

1. Heat pan add bacon and cook until bacon starts to become crispy. Add onion, garlic and mushrooms. Cook until mushrooms shrink and release moisture.
2. Add kale/spinach and cook until softened. Add dried herbs, salt and pepper and stir. Remove pan from heat.
3. Stir in cheese and set filling aside.

**Prepare the turkey:**

4. Place plastic wrap on top of each turkey breast and pound thinner into an even thickness, about 1/2-inch thick.
5. Place the turkey breast skin side down. Divide the filling between the tw turkey breasts. Fold one edge of turkey breast over and make into a roll. Tie turkey breast. Repeat with the other turkey breast.
6. Season top of tied breasts with additional salt and pepper. Coat air fryer basket with oil and then place the turkey skin-side down in the basket. (If you have a larger oven-style air fryer you'll be able to cook the two breasts at once (just make sure they aren't touching). However if you have a basket-style air fryer, you'll only be able to cook one breast at a time. Keep the second breast in the fridge until ready to cook.)
7. Air Fry at 360°F for 20 minutes. Flip the turkey breast to be skin-side up and Air Fry again for 10-20 minutes or until internal temperature of turkey reaches 165°F the thickest part. Allow to rest for 5 minutes and then slice and serve.

# Air Fryer Pork Tenderloin

**Cook Time: 26 minutes  Servings: 4**

## INGREDIENTS

- Pork tenderloin (1.25lbs – 1.75lbs)
- 2 tbs brown sugar
- 1 tbs smoked paprika
- 1.5 tsp salt
- 1 tsp ground mustard
- 1/2 tsp onion powder
- 1/2 tsp ground black pepper
- 1/4 tsp garlic powder
- 1/4 tsp cayenne powder (optional)
- 1/2 tbs olive oil

## DIRECTIONS

1. Mix all dry ingredients in a bowl.
2. Trim the pork tenderloin of any excess fat/silver skin. Coat with a 1/2 tablespoon olive oil. Rub spice mixture on entire pork tenderloin.
3. Preheat air fryer to 400° F for 5 minutes. After 5 minutes, carefully place pork tenderloin into air fryer and air fry at 400° F for 20-22 minutes. Internal temp should be 145° – 160° F.
4. When air fryer cycle is complete, carefully remove pork tenderloin to a cutting board and let rest for 5 minutes before slicing. Save any juices to serve over sliced meat.

◇◇◇◇◇◇◇◇◇◇◇◇◇◇◇◇◇◇◇◇◇◇◇◇◇◇◇◇◇◇◇◇◇◇◇◇◇◇◇◇◇

# Air Fryer Steak Bites

**Prep Time: 10 minutes  Cook Time: 18 minutes  Servings: 3**

## INGREDIENTS

- 1 lb. steaks , cut into 1/2" cubes (ribeye, sirloin, tri-tip or what you prefer)
- 8 oz. mushrooms (cleaned, washed and halved)
- 2 Tablespoons Butter , melted (or olive oil)
- 1 teaspoon Worcestershire sauce
- 1/2 teaspoon garlic powder , optional
- flakey salt , to taste
- fresh cracked black pepper , to taste
- Minced parsley , garnish
- Melted butter , for finishing - optional
- Chili Flakes , for finishing - optional

## DIRECTIONS

1. Rinse and thoroughly pat dry the steak cubes. Combine the steak cubes and mushrooms. Coat with the melted butter and then season with Worcestershire sauce, optional garlic powder, and a generous seasoning of salt and pepper.
2. Preheat the Air Fryer at 400°F for 4 minutes.
3. Spread the steak and mushrooms in an even layer in the air fryer basket. Air fry at 400°F for 10-18 minutes, shaking and flipping and the steak and mushrooms 2 times through cooking process (time depends on your preferred doneness, thickness of the steak, size of air fryer).
4. Check the steak to see how well done it is cooked. If you want the steak more done, add an extra 2-5 minutes of cooking time.
5. Garnish with parsley and drizzle with optional melted butter and/or optional chili flakes. Season with additional salt & pepper if desired. Serve warm.

# Chick-Fil-A Crispy Chicken Sandwich Copycat

**Prep Time: 30 minutes Cook Time: 10 minutes Servings: 4**

## INGREDIENTS

- 4 chicken breast halves
- 1/2 cup pickle juice
- 1/4 cup water
- 1/2 cup milk
- 1 large egg
- oil for frying
- 4 hamburger buns
- Pickle, lettuce, tomato and cheese slices , for topping

**For the breading:**

- 1 cup all-purpose flour
- 3 Tablespoons powdered sugar
- 1/2 teaspoon paprika
- 1 teaspoon freshly ground black pepper
- 1/2 teaspoon chili powder
- 1/2 teaspoon salt
- 1/2 teaspoon baking powder
- 1-2 teaspoons cayenne pepper *optional, for a spicy chicken sandwich

**For the Chick-fil-A-sauce**

- 1/2 cup mayonnaise
- 1 teaspoon dijon mustard
- 3 teaspoons yellow mustard
- 2 teaspoon barbecue sauce (hickory tastes the best)
- 2 Tablespoons honey
- 1/2 teaspoon garlic powder
- 1/2 teaspoon paprika
- 1 teaspoon lemon juice

## DIRECTIONS

1. Marinate the chicken: combine the pickle juice and water in a ziplock bag. Add the chicken breast halves and marinate for 30 minutes.
2. Make the sauce: Make the Chick-fil-A sauce by combining all ingredients in a bowl. Mix well and set aside.
3. Next, in a large bowl mix the breading ingredients together: flour, powdered sugar, paprika, black pepper, chili powder, salt, and baking powder.
4. In another bowl mix the milk, and egg.
5. Add 2-3 cups of oil to a large saucepan and heat oil to about 350 degrees F.
6. Coat the chicken: Dip the marinated chicken into the egg mixture, and then coat in the flour breading mixture. Now "double-dip" by repeating this step and dipping that same chicken tender back into the egg mixture and then back into the flour again!
7. Pan fry: Place chicken in hot oil and fry for 3-4 minutes on each side. Remove to paper towel to dry.
8. Assemble Sandwich: Toast the sandwich buns. Grab the Chick-fil-A sauce and smooth it on both sides of the buns. Top with lettuce, cheese, and crispy chicken! Enjoy!

# Air Fryer Chicken Parmesan

**Prep Time**: **10 minutes** **Cook Time**: **20 minutes** **Servings**: **4**

## INGREDIENTS

- 1 Lb Chicken Breast (about 4 small breasts)
- 1/4 Cup White whole wheat flour (or GF all purpose)
- 1/3 Cup Italian seasoned bread crumbs (GF if needed)
- 1/3 cup Italian seasoned Panko (GF if needed)
- 4 1/2 tsp Italian seasoning
- 3/4 tsp Salt
- 1/2 Cup + 2 Tbsp Parmesan Cheese, grated and divided
- 2 Large eggs
- 1/3 Cup Marinara sauce
- 1/2 Cup Mozzarella cheese, Grated
- Sliced basil, for garnish

## DIRECTIONS

1. Place the chicken between two layers of parchment paper and use a rolling pin or meat mallet to flatten about 1/2 inch thick.
2. Place the flour in a large, rimmed plate. Then, mix the bread crumbs, panko, Italian seasoning, salt, and 1/3 cup of the Parmesan cheese together and pour into another rimmed plate. Finally, whisk the eggs in a medium bowl.
3. Use one hand to dredge the chicken in the flour and then the egg, shaking off the excess. Use our other hand to cover the chicken in the panko mixture, pressing it on to coat it well. Place into the mesh air-fryer basket and repeat with all remaining chicken.
4. Bake at 400 degrees until the chicken starts to brown and get crispy, about 8-10 minutes.
5. Then, spread the marinara sauce on top of the chicken, followed by the rest of the Parmesan cheese and the mozzarella cheese. Bake for another 2-4 minutes, until the cheese is melted and the chicken reads 165 degrees F on the inside.
6. Sprinkle on basil and DEVOUR!

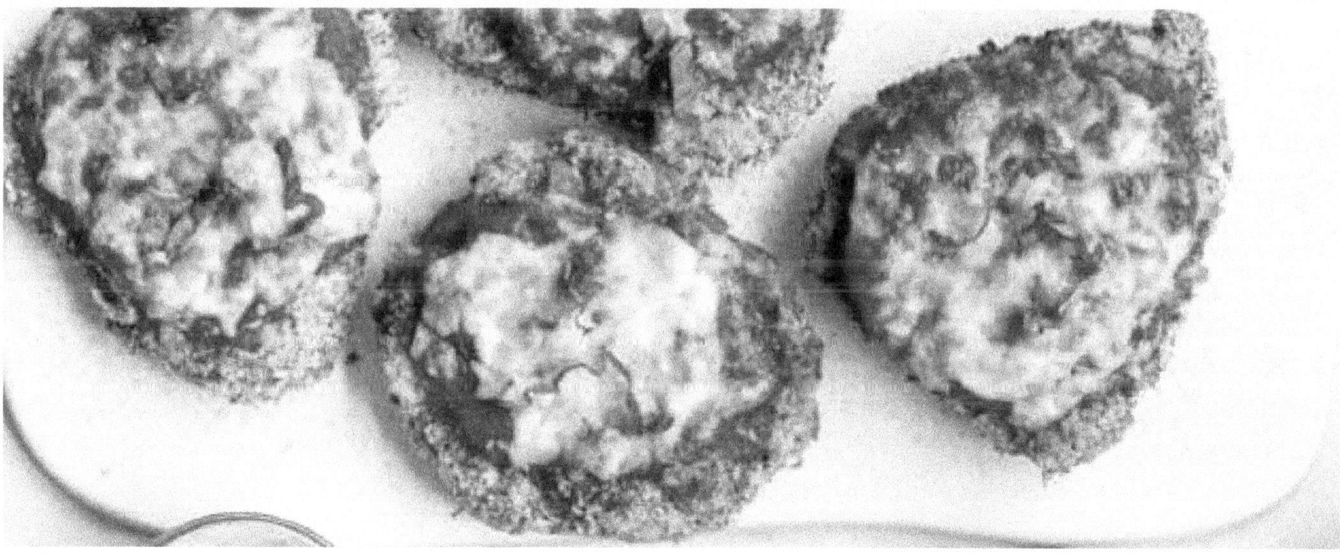

# Air Fryer Coconut Shrimp

**Prep Time: 20 minutes Cook Time: 20 minutes Servings: 4-5**

## INGREDIENTS

**coconut shrimp:**

- 1 ¼ pound jumbo raw shrimp (peeled + deveined)
- 1 cup EACH: shredded sweetened coconut AND Panko crumbs
- 1/3 cup all-purpose flour
- 2 large eggs
- ½ teaspoon EACH: garlic powder AND salt
- sweet and tangy sauce:
- 1/3 cup sweet chili sauce
- 2 teaspoons mayo
- ~ 1/2 lime, squeezed (more or less to taste)

## DIRECTIONS

1. PREP: Rinse the shrimp under cold running water, then, pat them dry on paper towels. Set up a dredging station. The first bowl should contain the flour, garlic powder, and ½ teaspoon of salt (whisk to combine.) In the second bowl, add the two eggs and whisk to combine. The third bowl will contain the shredded coconut and the Panko breadcrumbs, toss or stir to combine.
2. DREDGE: Grab the shrimp by the tail, dredge it in the flour, shake off any excess. Then, dip it in the egg mixture, and finally in the coconut mixture. Use your hands to press down so the crumbs adhere to the shrimp. Place the coated shrimp on a clean baking sheet. Continue with the remaining shrimp. At this point, you can freeze the shrimp for 30 minutes to make it easier to fry them or refrigerate until ready to fry. You can also fry or air fry them immediately.
3. COOK: FRY: Heat a large skillet over medium-high heat. Add a generous 1-1 ½ inches of oil tot he skillet and let it heat to about 350°F. Alternately, you could do this in a deep fryer set to 350°F. When heated, add a shrimp. Make sure the oil around the shrimp starts bubbling right away. Then, add 4-5 additional shrimp, make sure you do not overcrowd the pan. Cook for roughly 2 minutes per side (4-5 minutes total) or until the outside is golden brown and the shrimp curl up into a 'c' shape. Remove the shrimp with a slotted spoon and drain on a paper towel.
4. AIR FRYER: Preheat the air fryer according to manufacturers' directions at 375°F. Place the shrimp on a clean surface and spray the shrimp with coconut cooking spray (or any kind you like) place the sprayed side down in the air fryer and spray the other side with cooking spray. Cook the shrimp at 375°F for 6-8 minutes or until they cook all the way through, be sure to flip the shrimp around the halfway mark.
5. SAUCE: Combine the ingredients for the sauce in a bowl and whisk. You want to make sure to work the lumps out of the sauce completely. Taste and adjust with additional lime juice as desired. Serve with the shrimp!

# Crispy Peanut Tofu With Squash Noodles

**Prep Time**: **20 minutes** **Cook Time**: **20 minutes** **Servings**: **4**

## INGREDIENTS

**FOR THE PEANUT SAUCE:**

- 6 tablespoons powdered peanut butter I like PB2
- 1 clove garlic small, finely grated
- 1/2 teaspoon ginger paste
- 1 tablespoon low-sodium tamari or low-sodium soy sauce
- 1 teaspoon toasted sesame oil
- 1/2 teaspoon Chinese cooking wine

**FOR THE PEANUT TOFU AND SQUASH NOODLES:**

- 14 ounces extra firm tofu drained, pressed and diced into cubes
- 2 tablespoons low-sodium tamari or low-sodium soy sauce
- 1 teaspoon toasted sesame oil
- 1 tablespoon cornstarch
- 2 teaspoons toasted sesame seeds optional
- olive oil spray
- 2 medium yellow squash spiralized
- 2 medium zucchinis spiralized
- 6 to 8 ounces shiitake mushrooms stems removed and caps sliced
- 1/4 teaspoon garlic powder

**FOR SERVING:**

- 1/4 cup chopped peanuts for serving
- cilantro chopped, for serving
- 2 green onions sliced, for serving
- sambal oelek for serving
- lime wedges for serving
- sesame seeds for serving

## DIRECTIONS

**FOR THE SAUCE:**

1. In a small bowl, combine the powdered peanut butter with 3 tablespoons of water, mixing until combined.
2. Next stir in the garlic, ginger, tamari, toasted sesame oil and Chinese cooking wine.
3. When ready to serve, heat in a small sauce pan until warmed

**FOR THE TOFU AND SQUASH NOODLES:**

4. Cut the (pressed) tofu into ½-inch cubes.
5. In a medium bowl, combine 2 tablespoons tamari, 1 teaspoon sesame oil and cornstarch. Once combined, toss with sesame seeds.
6. Then, preheat your air fryer to 390° or 400° depending on your model. Working in batches, add the tofu in a single layer and air fry for 8 to 10 minutes or until crispy. Transfer to a paper towel lined plate and repeat with the remaining tofu.
7. Then add the sliced shiitake into the air fryer and cook for 4 minutes. You can reheat the tofu by adding it back into your air fryer and heating for a minute or two.

**FOR THE SQUASH NOODLES:**

8. Heat a 10-inch skillet over medium heat and spray with olive oil spray.
9. Once hot, add the spiralized squash noodles and the garlic powder. Toss occasionally until tender yet still a bit firm. About 7 to 8 minutes.
10. Finally serve the zoodles into bowls and add the crispy tofu, shiitake mushrooms and peanut sauce. Then top with crushed peanuts, sliced green onions, sesame seeds and minced cilantro. Don't forget about the wedge of lime on the side.

# Crunchy Air Fryer Fish

**Prep Time**: **5 minutes** **Cook Time**: **15 minutes** **Servings**: **4**

## INGREDIENTS

- 1 lb. white fish fillets (not more than ½ inch thick)
- 1 large egg
- ½ cup yellow cornmeal
- 1 tsp paprika
- ½ tsp garlic powder
- ½ tsp black pepper
- 1 tsp coarse salt
- oil spray
- lemon and parsley for garnish (Optional)

## DIRECTIONS

1. Preheat the air fryer for at least 3 minutes to 400 F. Whisk the egg in a shallow pan. In another shallow pan, combine the cornmeal and spices thoroughly.
2. Pat the fish completely dry. Dip the fish fillets into the egg - allow the excess to drip back into the pan. Then press the fish into the cornmeal mixture until well coated on both sides.
3. Place the coated fish into the preheated air fryer basket. Spritz lightly with oil. Cook for 10 minutes – stopping midway to flip the fish to ensure even cooking. If you notice dry spots, this is the time to spritz with a bit more oil. Return the basket to the air fryer and cook 5-7 minutes or until the fish is cooked through.
4. Once done, squeeze lightly with lemon and sprinkle with parsley or top with hot sauce as desired. Serve immediately.

◇◇◇◇◇◇◇◇◇◇◇◇◇◇◇◇◇◇◇◇◇◇◇◇◇◇◇◇◇◇◇◇◇◇◇◇◇◇◇◇◇◇

# Air Fryer Beef Tacos

**Prep Time: 15 minutes** **Cook Time: 20 minutes** **Servings**: **12**

## INGREDIENTS

- 1 lb ground beef
- salt and pepper
- 1 cup shredded mexican cheese
- 1-2 cups vegetable oil
- 12 yellow corn tortillas
- lettuce and tomato
- cooked cubed potatoes optional

## DIRECTIONS

1. Cook the ground beef until browned. Season with salt and pepper. Drain, if needed.
2. Add meat and shredded cheese to a bowl and mix. (add the optional potatoes)
3. In a large frying pan heat up 1-1.5 inches of vegetable oil.
4. Add about 1/3 cup of the meat mixture to the center of one tortilla. Fold the tortilla and clasp the top edges with tongs to keep it closed.
5. While holding the top of the tortilla place the bottom in the oil. Rock the tortilla from side to side a few times and then lie the tortilla on its side to fry.
6. Fry each side until golden brown and place on a plate lined with a paper towel to drain excess oil.
7. Fill each taco with lettuce and tomatoes before serving.

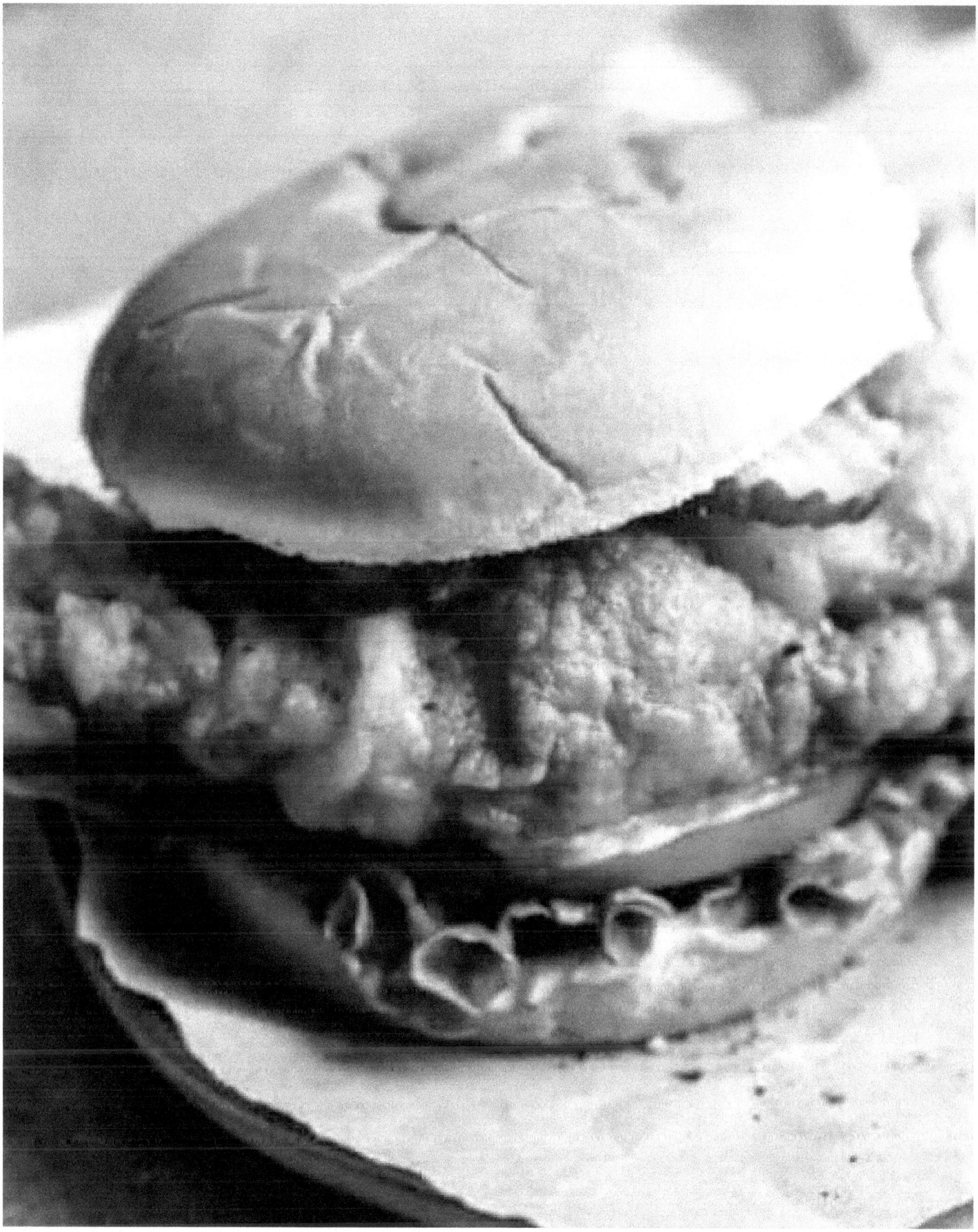

# Air Fryer Mozzarella Sticks

**Prep Time: 20 minutes    Servings: 4 - 6**

## INGREDIENTS

- 8 mozzarella string cheese sticks
- 3 large eggs
- 1 tbsp. water
- 1/2 c. breadcrumbs
- 1/2 c. panko breadcrumbs
- 1 tsp. Italian seasoning blend
- 1/4 tsp. garlic powder
- 1/4 tsp. smoked paprika
- 1/3 c. all-purpose flour
- 1/2 tsp. salt
- 1/4 tsp. ground black pepper
- Nonstick cooking spray
- Marinara sauce, to serve

## DIRECTIONS

1. Cut the cheese sticks in half, crosswise. Set aside.
2. Whisk together the eggs and water in a small bowl. In another small bowl, combine the breadcrumbs, panko, Italian seasoning, garlic powder, and paprika, stirring well. In a third bowl, combine the flour, salt, and pepper, stirring well.
3. Dip each of the cheese sticks into the eggs, then dredge in the flour mixture. Dip back into the eggs, then dredge in the bread crumb mixture, pressing to coat well.
4. Place the sticks on a small parchment-lined baking sheet. Freeze for 30 minutes. After 30 minutes, dip each of the sticks back into the eggs, then dredge in the breadcrumb mixture, pressing to coat well. Freeze again for 30 minutes.
5. Preheat the air fryer to 390°, if required. Spray the fryer basket with cooking spray. Generously coat the frozen sticks with cooking spray. In 2 batches, place the sticks in the basket in a single layer. Cook 6-7 minutes or until browned and crispy. (Keep an eye on them so they do not overcook or the cheese will start to bubble out.)
6. Serve immediately with warm marinara sauce.

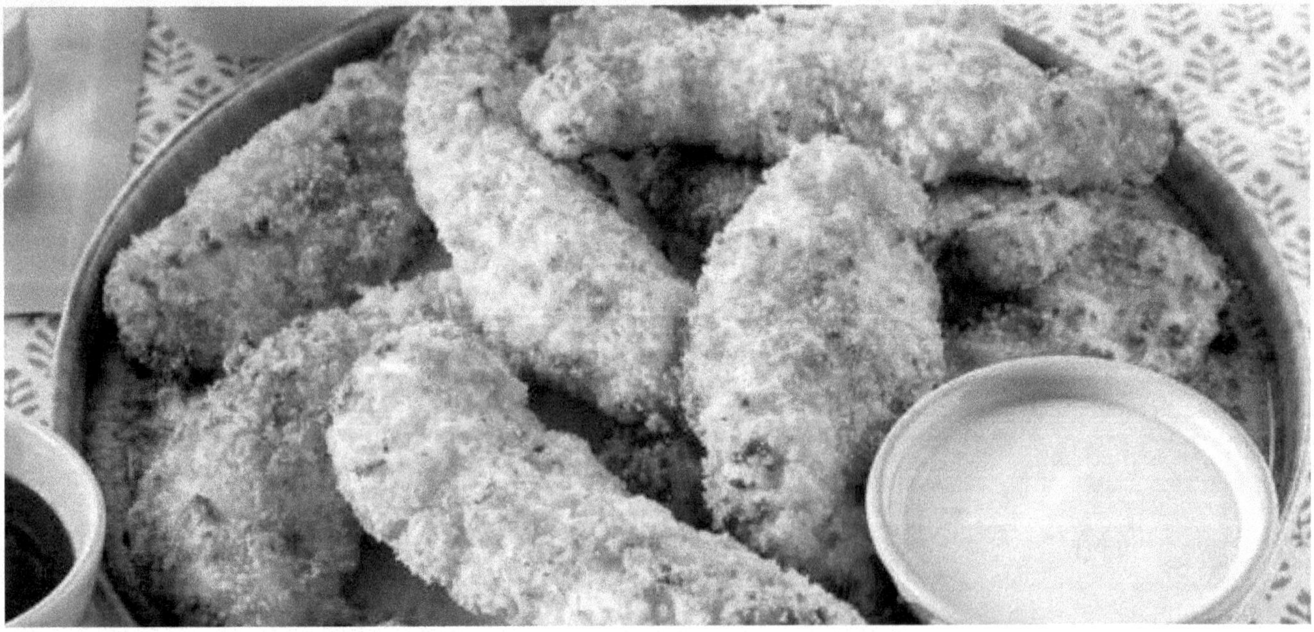

# Air Fryer Truffle Herb French Fries

**Prep Time: 15 minutes Cook Time: 35 minutes Resting Time: 10 minutes Servings: 2**

## INGREDIENTS

**SEARED STEAK**

- 2 strip steaks
- kosher salt
- freshly cracked black pepper
- 3 to 4 tablespoons unsalted butter

**TRUFFLE HERB FRIES IN THE AIR FRYER**

- 2 to 3 russet potatoes, thinly sliced
- olive oil for spritzing/brushing
- 1 teaspoon truffle salt
- 2 tablespoons chopped fresh parsley
- 2 tablespoons freshly grated parmesan cheese

**HONEY DIJON AIOLI**

- 1/3 cup mayonnaise
- 1 garlic clove, minced
- 1 tablespoon dijon mustard
- 2 teaspoons honey

## DIRECTIONS

**SEARED STEAK**

1. Make sure your steaks sit out at room temperature for about 30 minutes.
2. Heat a cast iron skillet over medium-high heat - you want it hot! Season the steaks on both sides with the salt and pepper.
3. Add 2 tablespoons of butter to the hot skillet. It will sizzle and smoke and once it's all melted, add in the steaks. Cook for 3 minute, until deeply golden, then flip and cook for 3 minutes more. Add in the remaining butter. Once it melts, spoon it over top of the steaks for another 1 to 2 minutes. I like to cook the steaks to about 140-145 degrees (almost medium doneness or medium well). Remove the steaks and let them rest for 10 to 15 minutes before slicing.

**TRUFFLE HERB FRIES IN THE AIR FRYER**

4. Place the sliced potatoes in a large bowl and cover with cold water. Let the potatoes sit in the water for 30 to 60 minutes. Remove the potatoes and place them on kitchen towels - you want them completely dry! Pat them as dry as you can!
5. Preheat your air fryer to 375 degrees F. Place the potatoes on a baking sheet and spray or brush with olive oil. Place the fries in a single layer in your air fryer (you might have to do 2 batches!). Cook for 12 minutes, then gently flip the fries and cook for 5 to 6 minutes more.
6. Stir together the parsley and parmesan cheese. When the fries are done, place them on a plate or a sheet of parchment paper and sprinkle all over with the truffle salt immediately. Sprinkle with the herbs and parmesan mixture. Serve with the aioli.
7. If you do 2 batches, or if the fries are done before the steak, you can stick these in a 200 degree F oven until ready to eat!

**HONEY DIJON AIOLI**

8. Whisk ingredients together until combined.

# Air Fryer Southwest Egg Rolls

**Prep Time: 15 minutes  Cook Time: 10 minutes  Servings: 6**

## INGREDIENTS

**Filling**

- 1 cup corn kernels frozen or canned (drained)
- 1 cup black beans rinsed and drained
- ½ cup finely diced red bell pepper
- ¼ cup finely diced jalapeno pepper
- ¼ cup chopped green onions
- 2 cups shredded chicken
- 3 cups shredded Monterey jack cheese
- 1 teaspoon paprika
- ½ teaspoon ground cumin
- 1 teaspoon mild chili powder
- ½ teaspoon salt
- Egg Rolls
- 1 egg
- 1 tablespoon water
- 12 egg roll wrappers
- Vegetable oil

**Zesty Dip**

- 1 cup sour cream or plain Greek yogurt
- ½ cup buttermilk ranch dressing or light ranch dressing
- 1 tablespoon taco seasoning

## DIRECTIONS

1. In a large mixing bowl, combine the corn, black beans, bell pepper, jalapenos, green onions, chicken, cheese and seasonings; set aside.
2. In a small bowl, use a fork to whisk together the egg and water.
3. Scoop ½ cup of the chicken mixture onto an egg roll wrapper. Brush the egg wash around the outside of the egg roll. Fold in two sides of the wrapper so the points almost touch. Then fold the top in and tightly roll up the egg roll and place on a sheet pan lined with waxed or parchment paper. Repeat with the remainder of the chicken mixture.
4. Lightly brush each egg roll with vegetable oil. Place egg rolls in an air fryer and cook at 375°F for 5 minutes. Make sure there is space between each egg roll - cook in batches if needed.
5. Use a tongs to flip the egg rolls and continue cooking for 3-5 more minutes or until the exterior is golden brown and crispy. (Cooking times can vary greatly depending on the brand and size of your air fryer. I did four at a time at 375°F and it took between 8-10 minutes total.)
6. While the egg rolls are in the air fryer, combine the sour cream, ranch dressing and taco seasoning to make the zesty dip. Refrigerate until ready to serve.

# Air Fryer Vegetarian Stuffed Peppers

**Prep Time**: **10 minutes** **Cook Time**: **15 minutes** **Servings**: **4**

## INGREDIENTS

- 4-6 Bell Peppers destemed and seeds removed
- 15 oz diced tomatoes
- 15 oz tomato sauce
- 1 cup cooked rice
- 1 can kidney beans drained and rinsed
- 1-2 T Italian Seasoning
- 1/2 cup mozzarella cheese
- 1 T parmesan cheese

## DIRECTIONS

1. Remove tops from bell peppers. Deseed and scoop them out. Take the tops (lids of bell peppers) and dice up.
2. Combine diced bell pepper tops, diced tomatoes (with juice), rice, beans and seasoning together.
3. Place mixture into scooped out bell peppers. Fill bell peppers almost to top with mixture.
4. Placed stuffed peppers into air fryer basket. Cook at 360 degrees F for 12 minutes. Remove from air fryer but keep in basket.
5. Top the air fryer stuffed peppers with cheese mixture and cook for another 3 minutes at 360 degrees F or until cheese is melted. ENJOY!

# Air Fryer Cauliflower Tacos

**Prep Time**: **15 minutes** **Cook Time**: **15 minutes** **Servings**: **12**

## INGREDIENTS

- 2 eggs
- 2 t chili powder
- 1 t cumin
- 1 cup panko bread crumbs I used a gluten-free kind
- 1 head cauliflower cut into bite sized florets
- oil spray - as needed
- 12 tortillas I used all corn
- Mango Salsa optional topping
- diced cabbage optional topping

## DIRECTIONS

1. In a bowl, whisk together the eggs and spices.
2. In another shallow bowl, put your bread crumbs.
3. Dredge one cauliflower floret at a time through the egg mixture and then into the bread crumbs. Once floret is fully covered place into air fryer basket. Be sure to put the vegetables in a single layer and not to over crowd within the basket.
4. Give the cauliflower florets a spritz of oil, if you wish. This will help the breading to crisp up. This step is optional.
5. Air fry the cauliflower bites at 350 degrees F for 14 minutes. At the 7 minute mark (half way through the cooking process) remove the air fryer basket and gently shake the veggie pieces.
6. When air fryer timer goes off, you can construct your tacos. Equally divide the air fried cauliflower pieces onto the 12 warmed tortillas. Top with your favorite toppings: I prefer diced purple cabbage and mango salsa.
7. ENJOY!

# Air Fryer Cheeseburgers

**Prep Time**: **5 minutes** **Cook Time**: **15 minutes** **Servings**: **4**

## INGREDIENTS

- 1 pound ground beef 80/20 mix of lean beef to fat must be kept cold
- 1 small yellow onion finely diced
- 1 clove garlic minced
- 2 teaspoons Worcestershire sauce
- Salt and pepper
- 4 Buns

## DIRECTIONS

1. Start by making the hamburger mix. In a mixing bowl, combine the ground beef with the garlic, onion, Worcestershire sauce, salt and pepper. Just fold in the other ingredients in the ground beef and make sure not to over mix the mixture.
2. Using your hands, quickly shape the hamburger patties and place on a tray. You want to make sure that the meat stays cold, because if you overwork the meat then the temperature of your hands will warm the meat up and that can result in really dense hamburgers. To shape the burgers, it's also a good idea to wet your hands a little as this will prevent the meat from sticking to your hands.
3. Preheat your air fryer to 395°F (200°C).
4. Lightly spray the air fryer basket with non-stick spray, and place your hamburger patties in the basket and cook to your desired doneness.
5. The best way to check for the doneness of the hamburger is by inserting a food thermometer in the center of the patty (see temperatures in notes below).
6. Now you're wondering how long are you going to air fry the hamburgers for. This depends on the thickness of your patties, but start with 12 minutes and keep checking until the hamburgers are cooking to your liking.
7. When the burgers are done, place cheese over each patty and the cheese will melt. This will result in a really delicious cheeseburger, and feel free to add more than just one slice of cheese if you like really 'cheesy' hamburgers just like my husband does!
8. Toast the buns in the air fryer on the same temperature, keep checking so that they're not burnt and just toasted.
9. Assemble the hamburgers and use your favorite toppings. I personally like mayonnaise, tomato slices, onion slices, and lettuce.

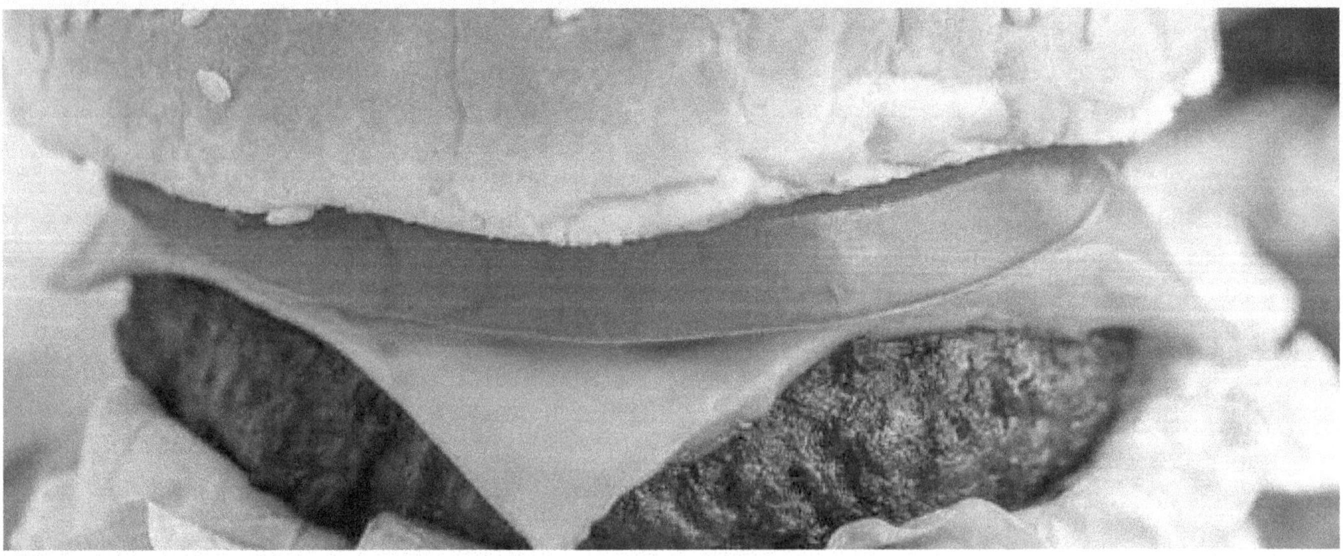

# Korean-Style Fried Cauliflower

**Prep Time: 20 minutes Cook Time: 40 minutes Servings: 4**

## INGREDIENTS

- 1 head cauliflower cut into bite-size florets (about 1 ½ pounds florets)
- 1 tablespoon cornstarch
- Pinch salt
- Pinch pepper
- Pinch baking powder

**BATTER:**

- 1 cup all-purpose flour
- ½ cup cornstarch
- 2 teaspoons baking powder
- 1 tablespoon garlic powder
- 1 cup cold water

**SAUCE:**

- 4 ½ tablespoons gochujang Korean chili sauce
- 4 tablespoons reduced sodium soy sauce
- 3 tablespoons honey
- 1 teaspoon sesame oil
- ½ teaspoon freshly grated ginger
- ½ teaspoon minced garlic
- ¼ teaspoon rice vinegar or apple cider vinegar
- Garnishes: lime zest sesame seeds, green onions, lime wedges, and/or Ranch dressing

## DIRECTIONS

1. In a small bowl, mix together 1 tablespoon cornstarch with a pinch each of salt, pepper, and baking powder. Sprinkle cauliflower florets with the mixture and stir to coat.
2. In a large bowl, whisk together the flour, cornstarch, baking powder, and garlic powder for the batter. Then add the cold water. The batter will be on the thick side, kind of like pancake batter.
3. Dip the cauliflower into the batter to coat, shake a little over the bowl to allow excess batter drip off, then place the coated cauliflower on a wire rack (with a paper towel underneath) to allow more excess batter to drip off. Better for excess to drip off before it goes into the air fryer.
4. Brush the air fryer basket with a light layer of oil to help reduce sticking. Place coated cauliflower into the air fryer basket in a single layer, with space between each floret. Cook at 350°F/177°C for 10-12 minutes, until parts are light golden brown. (For my air fryer, this took 4 batches to cook all cauliflower. Remove debris and re-coat basket with oil between each batch.)
5. While the cauliflower is cooking, you can finish dipping the remaining cauliflower florets, then work on the sauce. Whisk together the gochujang, soy sauce, honey, sesame oil, ginger, garlic, and vinegar in a small saucepan. Bring to a simmer over medium heat, then remove from heat.
6. Once cauliflower is done cooking, add it to a large bowl. Then pour the sauce over the cauliflower and gently stir to coat.
7. Serve immediately. If desired, garnish with lime zest, lime wedges, green onion, and sesame seeds. Delicious served with a side of Ranch dressing.

# Air Fryer Chicken Tenders

**Prep Time: 15 minutes Cook Time: 20 minutes Servings: 4 - 6**

## INGREDIENTS

- 2 lb. chicken tenders
- 1 c. buttermilk
- 1 1/2 tsp. seasoned salt, divided
- 3/4 tsp. black pepper, divided
- 1/2 c. all-purpose flour
- 2 eggs
- 2 c. panko breadcrumbs
- 1/2 c. freshly grated parmesan cheese (or 1/4 cup pre-grated parmesan cheese)
- Cooking spray, such as Pam Olive Oil
- Honey mustard, BBQ sauce, and/or ranch dressing, for serving

## DIRECTIONS

1. In a zip-top plastic bag, combine the chicken tenders, buttermilk, 1 teaspoon of seasoned salt and ½ teaspoon of black pepper. Seal and massage the buttermilk mixture into the tenders. Let marinate for 30 minutes, or up to 2 hours, in the refrigerator.
2. Meanwhile, place the flour on a small plate. In a wide shallow bowl, whisk together the two eggs. In another wide, shallow bowl, combine the panko, parmesan cheese, remaining 1/2 teaspoon of seasoned salt and 1/4 teaspoon of black pepper.
3. Using a pair of tongs, remove the chicken from the buttermilk marinade (reserve the marinade) and place the chicken in a single layer on a paper-towel lined plate. Pour the remaining buttermilk marinade into the bowl with the eggs and whisk to combine.
4. Working 2-3 tenders at a time, dredge all over in the flour, dip in the egg mixture to coat completely, then dredge to coat completely in the panko breadcrumb mixture. Repeat until all of the tenders are breaded. Spray all over both sides of each tender with cooking spray (olive oil spray gives great flavor!)
5. Working in two batches, place the tenders in a single layer, with about ½-inch of space between them. Cook in the air fryer set at 380°F for 8 minutes. Then flip and continue to cook for 4-6 minutes longer, until the internal temperature of the chicken reads 165°F. Repeat with the second batch of tenders. Serve immediately alongside dipping sauces such as honey mustard, BBQ sauce, and/or ranch dressing.

# Air Fryer Brussels Sprouts

**Prep Time: 5 minutes    Servings: 3 - 4**

## INGREDIENTS

- 1 lb. Brussels sprouts
- 1 tbsp. olive oil
- 1/2 tsp. salt
- 1/4 tsp. ground black pepper
- 1 tbsp. soy sauce
- 2 tsp. honey
- 1/2 tsp. sriracha or chili-garlic sauce
- Salt & pepper, for serving

## DIRECTIONS

1. Heat an air fryer to 380 degrees. Trim the ends of the Brussels sprouts, keeping the roots intact, then cut in half through the root.
2. In a large bowl, combine the Brussels sprouts, olive oil, salt and pepper.
3. Place the Brussels sprouts in the basket and cook for 8 minutes. Remove the basket and shake the sprouts. Return to the air fryer for 8-10 more minutes, until crispy on the outside and tender on the inside.
4. Meanwhile, in the same large bowl, whisk to combine the soy sauce, honey and sriracha. Add the cooked Brussels sprouts back into this bowl and toss to coat. Season with additional salt and pepper, if desired, and serve immediately.
5. This content is created and maintained by a third party, and imported onto this page to help users provide their email addresses. You may be able to find more information about this and similar content at piano.io

◇◇◇◇◇◇◇◇◇◇◇◇◇◇◇◇◇◇◇◇◇◇◇◇◇◇◇◇◇◇◇◇◇◇◇◇◇◇◇◇

# Air Fryer Zucchini Corn Fritters

**Prep Time: 10 minutes    Cook Time: 12 minutes    Servings: 4**

## INGREDIENTS

- 2 medium zucchini
- 1 cup corn kernels
- 1 medium potato cooked
- 2 tbsp chickpea flour
- 2-3 garlic finely minced
- 1-2 tsp olive oil
- salt and pepper

**For Serving:**

- Ketchup or Yogurt tahini sauce

## DIRECTIONS

1. Grate zucchini using a grater or food processor. In a mixing bowl, mix grated zucchini with a little salt and leave it for 10-15 min. Then squeeze out excess water from the zucchini using clean hands or using a cheesecloth.
2. Also, grate or mash the cooked potato*.
3. Combine zucchini, potato, corn, chickpea flour, garlic, salt, and pepper in a mixing bowl.
4. Roughly take 2 tbsp batter, give it a shape of a patty and place them on parchment paper**.
5. Lightly brush oil on the surface of each fritter. Preheat Air Fryer to 360F.
6. Place the fritters on the preheated Air Fryer mesh without touching each other. Cook them for 8 min.
7. Then turn the fritters and cook for another 3 4 min or until well done or till you get the desired color.
8. Serve warm with ketchup or yogurt tahini sauce (see notes to prepare)

# Air Fryer Honey Mustard Salmon

**Prep Time: 5 minutes Cook Time: 10 minutes Servings: 3**

## INGREDIENTS

- 3 salmon fillets 1 ½ inches thick
- salt and pepper
- 2 tablespoons honey
- 1 tablespoon Dijon mustard

## DIRECTIONS

1. Make a foil sling for the air fryer basket, about 4 inches tall and a few inches longer than the width of the basket. Lay foil widthwise across basket, pressing it into and up the sides. Lightly spray foil and basket with cooking spray.
2. Pat salmon dry with paper towels. Season with salt and pepper.
3. In a small bowl, mix together honey and Dijon, until well combined. Reserve 1 tablespoon of glaze. Drizzle remaining glaze evenly over salmon fillets, tops and sides.
4. Arrange fillets skin side down on sling in the basket, with space between them. (The number of fillets you can fit in your air fryer at one time depends on the size of the fillets and the size of your air fryer.)
5. Cook at 350°F/175°C for 8-10 minutes, until salmon flakes easily and registers at 145°F/62.8°C (thinner salmon will be ready sooner, thicker salmon will take more time).
6. Using sling, carefully lift salmon from air fryer. Loosen the skin with a fish spatula or utensil, then transfer fillets to plate, leaving skin behind.
7. Drizzle reserved sauce over fillets. Garnish with fresh parsley, if desired. Serve warm.

◇◇◇◇◇◇◇◇◇◇◇◇◇◇◇◇◇◇◇◇◇◇◇◇◇◇◇◇◇◇◇◇◇◇◇◇◇◇◇◇

# Air Fryer Bacon-Wrapped Steak

**Prep Time: 15 minutes Cook Time: 18 minutes Servings: 4**

## INGREDIENTS

- 2 steaks rib eye steaks are best
- 6 strips bacon if you choose to wrap them
- 1 tbsp salt coarse ground
- 1/4 tsp chili powder
- 1/4 tsp pepper
- 1 tsp garlic powder
- 1/2 tsp onion powder

## DIRECTIONS

1. Mix seasonings together until combined well.
2. Lay steaks on cutting board and sprinkle half seasoning mix on 1 side of both steaks, pat down so it sticks. Flip over and do the same until seasonings are gone.
3. Lay 3 pieces of bacon down horizontally, lined up next to one another but not overlapping.
4. Lay 1 steak on top of the bacon in the middle. Wrap top piece around and under steak. Do this with 2nd piece, then with 3rd piece pull last side up and tuck it under one of the other pieces of bacon so they don't all unravel.
5. Do the same for your 2nd steak. Lay both bacon wrapped steaks inside your air fryer basket.
6. Preheat your air fryer at 375 degrees for 5 minutes, then put basket with steaks inside and set for a total of 18 minutes.
7. After 9 minutes flip both steaks so other side can cook and crisp bacon.
8. Allow steaks to rest for 3-5 minutes to stay juicy, then serve.

# Air-Fried Buffalo Cauliflower Bites

**Prep Time: 15 minutes    Cook Time: 30 minutes    Servings: 5**

## INGREDIENTS

- 1 large head cauliflower, cut into 1½-inch florets
- 8 tbsp. melted butter
- 1/2 c. cayenne pepper sauce (like Frank's Wing Sauce), plus more for dipping
- 1 1/2 c. almond flour or breadcrumbs
- 2 tsp. no-salt seasoning (optional)
- 1 c. ranch dressing, for dipping or as needed

## DIRECTIONS

1. Preheat the oven to the lowest temperature and then turn it off. Alternatively, turn it to a "keep warm" setting.
2. Place the cauliflower florets in a large bowl.
3. In a small bowl, mix the melted butter and cayenne pepper sauce to combine, then pour the sauce over the cauliflower. Mix everything together well.
4. In a separate large bowl or large resealable plastic bag, combine the almond flour or breadcrumbs and seasoning (if using). Transfer the cauliflower to the bowl or bag with the breading. Use tongs or a slotted spoon so you don't end up pouring in extra sauce. Toss (or shake) the cauliflower to coat it in the breading.
5. Transfer half of the coated cauliflower to your air fryer, using both the bottom and upper racks to avoid overcrowding.
6. Set the air fryer to 350° and cook for 12 to 15 minutes, until the cauliflower is golden brown and cooked through, but not mushy.
7. Place the cooked cauliflower on a sheet pan in the oven to keep warm. Continue to cook the remaining cauliflower in the air fryer.
8. To make the buffalo ranch dipping sauce, add your desired amount of wing sauce to the ranch dressing, to taste. Serve the buffalo cauliflower with the dipping sauce.

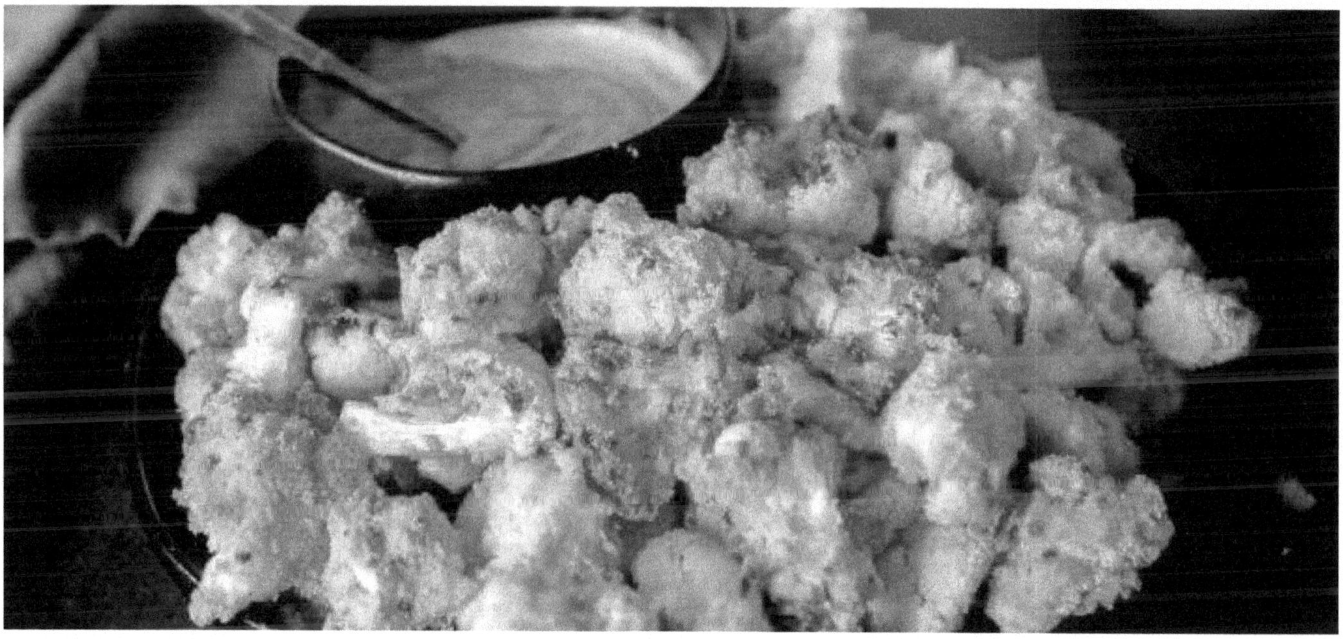

# Air Fryer Egg Fried Rice

**Prep Time**: **5 minutes** **Cook Time**: **15 minutes** **Servings**: **4**

## INGREDIENTS

- 3 c rice cooked and cold
- 1 c frozen vegetables I used carrot, corn, broccoli and edamame
- 1/3 c coconut aminos
- 1 T oil
- 2 eggs scrambled (optional)

## DIRECTIONS

1. To make your air fryer fried rice, put your cold rice into an large bowl.
2. Then add your frozen vegetables to the rice bowl.
3. If you are using egg or another protein, add it to the rice bowl now.
4. Next up, you are going to add the coconut aminos and oil to your bowl.
5. Mix, mix, mix until well combined. Then transfer to the rice mixture to an oven safe container.
6. Place that container into your air fryer. Cook the air fryer fried rice at 360 degrees F for 15 minutes. I would suggest stirring 3 times through the 15 minutes.
7. Enjoy!

◇◇◇◇◇◇◇◇◇◇◇◇◇◇◇◇◇◇◇◇◇◇◇◇◇◇◇◇◇◇◇◇◇◇◇◇◇◇◇◇

# Air Fryer Cheesy Cauliflower Arancini

**Prep Time: 30 minutes** **Cook Time: 10 minutes** **Servings: 12**

## INGREDIENTS

- 2 italian chicken sausage links, any casing removed
- 4 ½ cups frozen cauliflower rice
- ½ teaspoon salt
- 1 ½ cups marinara sauce
- 1 cup freshly grated mozzarella cheese
- olive oil spray for spritzing
- 2 large eggs
- ½ cup seasoned bread crumbs
- 2 tablespoons freshly grated parmesan cheese

## DIRECTIONS

1. Heat a large skillet over medium high heat. Add the sausage and cook it, breaking it apart with a spoon until it's in small crumbles. Cook for about 4 to 5 minutes.
2. Stir in the cauliflower rice, salt, and ½ cup of the marinara sauce. Cook the mixture over medium heat, stirring often, until the cauliflower is tender, about 6 to 8 minutes. Remove the skillet from the heat and let it cool for 5 minutes, then stir in the mozzarella cheese. Let the mixture cool slightly until it's easy to handle.
3. Scoop out ¼ cup of the mixture and form it into a ball with your hands. Place the ball on a baking sheet. Repeat this with the remaining cauliflower mixture.
4. Lightly beat the eggs in a small bowl. In another bowl, stir together the bread crumbs and grated parmesan. Take each ball and lightly dip it in the egg mixture, then roll it through the bread crumbs to coat it completely. Repeat with the remaining balls.
5. Once all the arncini are made, preheat the air fryer to 400 degrees. Spray the arancini with the cooking spray all over - this really helps to crisp them up! Once the air fryer is heated, add the arancini in the basket (you may need to do 2 batches) and cook for 9 to 10 minutes, gently flipping the arancini half way through.
6. Heat the remaining marinara sauce and serve the arancini with it immediately for dipping.

# Air Fryer Omelette

**Cook Time: 8 minutes**

**INGREDIENTS**

- 2 eggs
- 1/4 cup milk
- Pinch of salt
- Fresh meat and veggies, diced (I used red bell pepper, green onions, ham and mushrooms)
- 1 teaspoon McCormick Good Morning Breakfast Seasoning – Garden Herb
- 1/4 cup shredded cheese (I used cheddar and mozzarella)

**DIRECTIONS**

1. In a small bowl, mix the eggs and milk until well combined.
2. Add a pinch of salt to the egg mixture.
3. Add your veggies to the egg mixture.
4. Pour the egg mixture into a well-greased 6″x3″ pan.
5. Place the pan into the basket of the air fryer.
6. Cook at 350° Fahrenheit for 8-10 minutes.
7. Halfway through cooking sprinkle the breakfast seasoning onto the eggs and sprinkle the cheese over the top.
8. Use a thin spatula to loosen the omelette from the sides of the pan and transfer to a plate.
9. Garnish with extra green onions, optional

# Air Fryer Cheesy Chicken Dinner

**Prep Time: 10 minutes Cook Time: 8 minutes Servings: 4**

**INGREDIENTS**

- 4 thin chicken breasts or two chicken breasts cut/pounded to be thin
- 1 cup milk
- [1/2 cup panko bread crumbs]
- 3/4-1 cup shaved Parmesan-Asiago cheese blend can use any type of hard shaved or shredded cheese like Parmesan, Asiago, Romano
- salt + pepper to taste

**DIRECTIONS**

1. Preheat your air fryer to 400 degrees. Spray the cooking basket lightly with cooking spray.
2. In a large bowl place the milk and chicken breasts. Sprinkle in a generous pinch of salt and freshly ground pepper. Allow to marinate in the milk for 10 minutes.
3. In a shallow bowl combine panko bread crumbs and shaved cheese.
4. Dredge chicken breasts through panko and cheese mixture (press the mixture on top of the chicken generously) and place in the air fryer basket. Make sure that the basket is not overcrowded. I fit 2 chicken breasts in the basket, so I did this in two batches. Spray the top of the chicken lightly with cooking spray (this 'locks on' the cheesy bread crumb topping).
5. Cook for 8 minutes, flipping the chicken breasts halfway through.
6. Remove from the air fryer, repeat the process with any remaining chicken breasts. If you want to warm everything, you can add the already cooked chicken breasts into the basket and cook them for 1 minute to warm them! Enjoy

# Air Fryer Brazilian-Style Drumsticks

**Prep Time**: **5 minutes** **Cook Time**: **25 minutes** **Marinating Time**: **30 minutes** **Servings**: **4**

## INGREDIENTS

- 1 teaspoon cumin seeds
- 1 teaspoon dried oregano
- 1 teaspoon dried parsley
- 1 teaspoon ground turmeric
- 1/2 teaspoon coriander seeds
- 1 teaspoon kosher salt
- 1/2 teaspoon black peppercorns
- 1/2 teaspoon cayenne pepper
- 1/4 cup fresh lime juice
- 2 tablespoons olive oil
- 1 1/2 pounds chicken drumsticks

## DIRECTIONS

**MAKE THE MARINADE:**

1. In a clean coffee grinder or spice mill, combine the cumin, oregano, parsley, turmeric, coriander seeds, salt, peppercorns and cayenne pepper. Process until finely ground
2. In a small bowl, combine the ground spices with lime juice and oil. Place the chicken in a resealable bag. Add the marinade, seal and massage until the chicken is well coated. Marinate at room temperature for 30 minutes or in the refrigerator for up to 24 hours.
3. When you are ready to cook, place the drumsticks, skin side up in the air fryer basket. Set the airfryer to 400° for 20-25 minutes, turning the legs halfway through the cooking time. Use a meat thermometer to ensure that the chicken has reached an internal temperature of 165°.
4. Serve with plenty of napkins.

◇◇◇◇◇◇◇◇◇◇◇◇◇◇◇◇◇◇◇◇◇◇◇◇◇◇◇◇◇◇◇◇◇◇◇◇◇◇◇◇

# Air Fryer Breakfast Burritos

**Prep Time**: **15 minutes** **Cook Time**: **5 minutes** **Servings**: **6**

## INGREDIENTS

- 6 medium flour tortillas
- 6 scrambled eggs
- 1/2 lb ground sausage – browned
- 1/2 bell pepper – minced
- 1/3 cup bacon bits
- 1/2 cup shredded cheese
- oil for spraying

## DIRECTIONS

1. Combine scrambled eggs, cooked sausage, bell pepper, bacon bits & cheese in a large bowl. Stir to combine.
2. Spoon about 1/2 cup of the mixture into the center of a flour tortilla.
3. Fold in the sides & then roll.
4. Repeat with remaining ingredients.
5. Place filled burritos into the air fryer basket & spray liberally with oil.
6. Cook at 330 degrees for 5 minutes.

# Air Fryer Crispy Cod

**Prep Time: 5 minutes  Cook Time: 12 minutes  Servings: 2**

**INGREDIENTS**

- 1 lb cod fillet
- 1 lemon
- 1/4 cup butter
- 1 tsp salt
- 1 tsp seasoning salt

**DIRECTIONS**

1. Prepare ingredients for the air fryer cod fillets. Season fillets with your favorite seasoning.
2. Brush the air fryer basket with oil. Place fillets in the basket. Top it off with butter and lemon slices.
3. Cook cod in the air fryer at 400 °F for 10-13 minutes, depending on the size of fillets. The internal temperature should reach 145 °F.

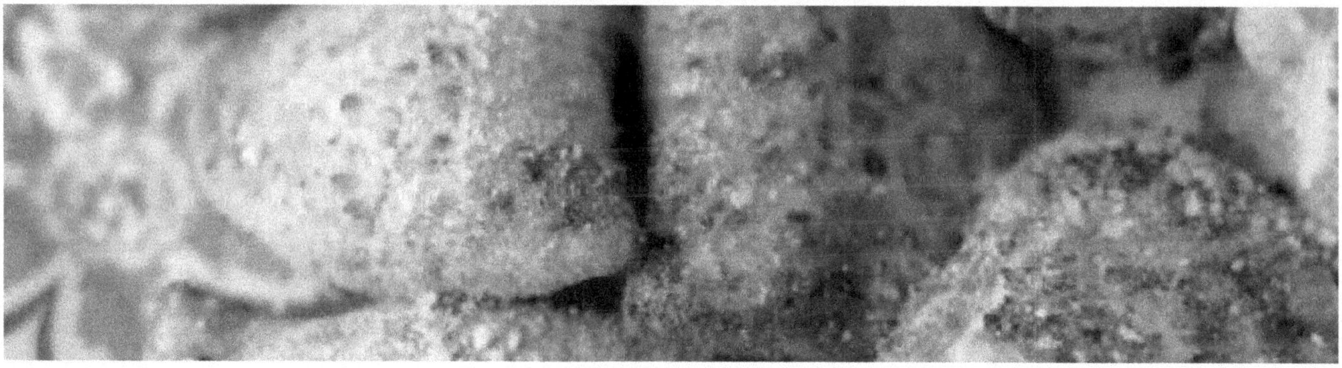

# Air Fryer Toasted Pierogies

**Prep Time: 15 minutes  Cook Time: 12 minutes  Servings: 6**

**INGREDIENTS**

- 1 bag store bought frozen Perogies
- 2 cups Italian-style bread crumbs
- 1 egg
- 1 cup buttermilk
- Olive Oil Spray
- Parmesan cheese optional

**DIRECTIONS**

1. Whisk together egg and buttermilk. Dip Perogi in the egg/milk mixture and then cover with breadcrumbs. Repeat with all perogies.
2. Add perogies to the air fryer basket and spray with olive oil spray. Close the fryer basket and press power. Set the temperature to 400 degrees F and time to 12 minutes. Halfway through, pause and turn the perogies over. Add additional spray, if needed.
3. Garnish with additional Parmesan cheese and serve hot.

## Cinnamon-Sugar Air Fryer Doughnuts

**Prep Time: 10 minutes  Cook Time: 5 minutes  Servings: 8**

**INGREDIENTS**

- 16 oz refrigerated flaky jumbo biscuits
- 1/2 c. granulated white sugar
- 2 tsp ground cinnamon
- 4 Tbsp butter melted
- olive or coconut oil spray

**DIRECTIONS**

1. Combine sugar and cinnamon in a shallow bowl; set aside.
2. Remove the biscuits from the can, separate them and place them on a flat surface. Use a 1-inch round biscuit cutter (or similarly-sized bottle cap) to cut holes out of the center of each biscuit.
3. Lightly coat air fryer basket with olive or coconut oil spray. Do not use non-stick spray like Pam because it can damage the coating on the basket.
4. Place 4 donuts in a single layer in the air fryer basket. Make sure they are not touching.
5. Air Fry at 360 degrees F for 5 minutes or until lightly browned.
6. Remove donuts from Air Fryer, dip in melted butter then roll in cinnamon sugar to coat. Serve immediately.

◇◇◇◇◇◇◇◇◇◇◇◇◇◇◇◇◇◇◇◇◇◇◇◇◇◇◇◇◇◇◇◇◇◇◇◇◇◇◇◇◇

## Air Fryer Sausage Rolls

**Prep Time: 5 minutes  Cook Time: 10 minutes  Servings: 12**

**INGREDIENTS**

- Air Fryer Sausage Rolls
- 3 sausages Note 1
- 3 sheets puff pastry
- 1 tbsp sesame seeds
- 1 eggs

**DIRECTIONS**

1. Air Fryer Sausage Rolls
2. Turn the air fryer on to 180°C/350 F for 15 minutes
3. Use a knife and chopping board to remove the casing from the sausages
4. Add egg to a small bowl, pierce yoke and whisk
5. Place a sheet of puff pastry (thawed) onto the chopping board and place 1 off the sausages on top
6. Roll the pastry around the sausage, then use a pastry brush to coat the top of the pastry where the 2 bits of pastry will meet
7. Continue to roll the pastry around the sausage and again brush one side of where the pastry joins with the egg
8. Repeat for each sausage
9. Brush the top of the length of the long rolled sausage with egg
10. Sprinkle the top with sesame seeds
11. Use a knife to cut the excess pastry off each end
12. Then cut the long sausage roll into 4 smaller rolls
13. Spray the Air Fryer Basket with oil (or use baking paper) then place raw sausage rolls into Air Fryer (work in batches)
14. Cook sausage rolls in Air Fryer for 7- 9 minutes until pastry is golden and crispy
15. Serve with sauce

# Air Fryer Loaded Breakfast Egg Rolls

**Prep Time: 30 minutes Cook Time: 20 minutes Servings: 18-20**

## INGREDIENTS

- 2 tablespoons unsalted butter
- 1 lb breakfast sausage
- 1 teaspoons kosher salt, divided
- 1 teaspoon fresh ground black pepper, divided
- 1/2 teaspoon garlic powder
- 1 small russet potato, finely grated
- 6 large Pete and Gerry's® Organic Eggs, lightly scrambled
- 18–20 egg roll wrappers
- 1 1/4 cup shredded sharp cheddar cheese
- 4 slices of bacon, cooked and chopped
- 1 small avocado, finely chopped
- Vegetable oil, for frying

## DIRECTIONS

1. Melt butter in a large skillet (preferably cast-iron) over medium heat. Once melted, add in sausage and let sausage brown and cook through completely, about 5-6 minutes. Season sausage with 1/2 teaspoon of salt/pepper and garlic powder.
2. Move sausage over to one side of skillet and add in potatoes. Let lightly cook and brown for about 2-3 minutes. Then mix with sausage and continue cooking for another 2-3 minutes. Once potatoes are lightly crisp, move mixture over to one side of skillet again.
3. Scramble eggs in a bowl with remaining 1/2 teaspoon of salt/pepper. Pour into empty side of skillet and lightly scramble for 1 minute. Then combine fully with sausage/potato mixture. At this stage you're looking for eggs to be lightly done- they do not need to be fully cooked as they will finish cooking when frying. Remove filling from heat and allow to cool down completely.
4. To make egg roll: Fill a small bowl with water and set aside. Wet your fingers with water and run them along the sides of egg roll wrapper. Place 2-3 tablespoons of filling directly into the center. Sprinkle top of filling with about a tablespoon of cheese, and a sprinkle of bacon and avocado. Bring the egg roll wrapper sides in and begin to roll up the egg roll all while tucking the filling in as you roll. Use more water once you get to the top if needed to seal completely. The key is to roll the egg rolls tightly without any exposed pockets. Then place egg rolls onto a small baking sheet. Repeat process until all wrappers are filled/rolled.
5. To fry: If using a traditional deep fryer: fill with oil and fry egg rolls, in batches, according to manufacturer's instructions- about 3-4 minutes or until golden brown and crispy. Then set aside on baking sheet with paper towel to blot excess oil. If using stovetop method: fill a large heavy-bottomed pot/dutch oven halfway with oil and use a deep fry thermometer to bring oil up to 360-370°F. Once that temperature is achieved, fry egg rolls, in batches, about 3-4 minutes or until golden brown and crispy. Then set aside on baking sheet with paper towel to blot excess oil.
6. Serve the egg rolls immediately with salsa, ketchup, or as desired. Enjoy!

# Air Fryer Italian Pork Chops

**Prep Time: 10 minutes Cook Time: 18 minutes Servings: 3**

**INGREDIENTS**

- 3 (6 oz.) ((170g)) pork chops , rinsed & patted dry
- salt , to taste
- black pepper , to taste
- garlic powder , to taste
- smoked paprika , to taste
- 1/2 cup (54 g) breadcrumbs , approximately
- 1/2 cup (50 g) grated parmesan cheese
- 2 Tablespoons (30 ml) chopped Italian parsley , plus more for optional garnish
- 1 large egg
- Cooking spray , for coating the pork chops
- 1/2 cup (56 g) grated mozzarella cheese
- 1 cup (240 ml) marinara sauce , heated

**DIRECTIONS**

1. Season the pork chops with salt, pepper, garlic powder, and smoked paprika. In medium bowl, mix together the breadcrumbs, parmesan cheese, and chopped parsley. In another bowl, beat the egg.
2. Dip each pork chop in egg and then dredge it in the breadcrumb mixture, coating completely. Lightly spray both sides of coated pork chops with cooking spray right before cooking.
3. Preheat the Air Fryer at 380°F for 4 minutes.
4. Place in the Air Fryer and cook at 380°F (194°C) for 8-12 minutes.
5. After 6 minutes of cooking, flip the pork chops and then continue cooking for the remainder of time or until golden and internal temperature reaches 145-160°F. Top with cheese and air fry for 2 more minutes to melt the cheese. Serve warm with marinara sauce.

# Air Fryer Chicken and Veggies

**Prep Time: 5 minutes Cook Time: 15 minutes Servings: 4**

**INGREDIENTS**

- 1 pound chicken breast, chopped into bite-size pieces (2-3 medium chicken breasts)
- 1 cup broccoli florets (fresh or frozen)
- 1 zucchini chopped
- 1 cup bell pepper chopped (any colors you like)
- 1/2 onion chopped
- 2 cloved garlic minced or crushed
- 2 tablespoons olive oil
- 1/2 teaspoon EACH garlic powder, chili powder, salt, pepper
- 1 tablespoon Italian seasoning (or spice blend of choice)

**DIRECTIONS**

1. Preheat air fryer to 400F.
2. Chop the veggies and chicken into small bite-size pieces and transfer to a large mixing bowl.
3. Add the oil and seasoning to the bowl and toss to combine.
4. Add the chicken and veggies to the preheated air fryer and cook for 10 minutes, shaking halfway, or until the chicken and veggies are charred and chicken is cooked through. If your air fryer is small, you may have to cook them in 2-3 batches.

CPSIA information can be obtained
at www.ICGtesting.com
Printed in the USA
LVHW060119010522
717630LV00011B/649